Top 20 Diets for Weight Loss

A Guide to The Top-Ranked Diets Plus a 7-Day Meal Plan to Get Started for a Healthier, More Energized, and Slimmer You

Yara Green

Dawn Publishing House

contained within this document, including, but not limited to, errors, omissions, or inaccuracies.

Table of Contents

Introduction

So many people struggle with their weight because they feel they have to eat a certain way and deprive themselves of what they like in order for the excess weight to come off. What ends up happening is people give up on changing their diet because it isn't sustainable and find themselves binging more than making better food choices. This is why fad diets gain overnight popularity. These types of diets promise rapid weight loss in a few short weeks but they never disclose how quickly the weight comes back. Instead of trying another fad diet that will only lead to disappointment, why not approach dieting as a new way of eating? Not a temporary fix but a long term solution. There are plenty of diets you can choose from that will allow you to easily lose weight and keep it off.

This book outlines the best diets for weight loss and better health. Each chapter will focus on a specific diet: what it is, what to eat, and how it works. No diet comes without setbacks. Each chapter also includes an overview of the drawbacks you may experience when transitioning to a new plan. These cons will help you determine if a diet is something you can maintain long-term.

You will also find a seven day meal plan at the end of each chapter. These options will help you see how versatile your meals can be week to week. The meal plans are designed to cater to each specific diet; some will have three meals outlined while others will have snacks and desserts included. Each meal plan can be modified to suit your lifestyle. While each plan provides multiple options for breakfast, lunch, and dinner, it is not realistic to expect you to cook a new meal three times a day. Instead, consider using leftovers for lunches or plan a leftover night one day a week to use up some of the food you have in your fridge.

Feel free to look over the meal plans in each chapter, even if you are not interested in starting a particular diet. Most of the meals can be used with any plan. For example, most Atkin's meals can be used with a low-carb diet. Most Mediterranean meals can be used with a whole-foods plant-based diet or a flexitarian diet, with slight modifications.

Stop trying to figure out why you can't lose weight or which diet will help you achieve your ideal weight. Find the right diet for you that you can stick with long-term so you can feel good about yourself for the rest of your life. If you are ready to get started with your new healthy eating habits let's take a look at the 20 best options for you to choose from.

Chapter 1:

The Atkins Diet

The Atkins diet is one of the most well-known low-carb diets. It gained popularity in the 1990s because of its promise of rapid weight loss after just two weeks. When celebrities like Jennifer Aniston, Alyssa Milano, and even Kim Kardashian endorsed the Atkins Diet, many people wanted to eat like them. While the popularity of the original Atkins diet has died down, other low-carb diets have gained popularity because of it. The Atkins diet has many benefits and is well-structured for both weight loss and better health. In this chapter, you will learn if the Atkins diet is right for you and how you can begin on a low-carb diet.

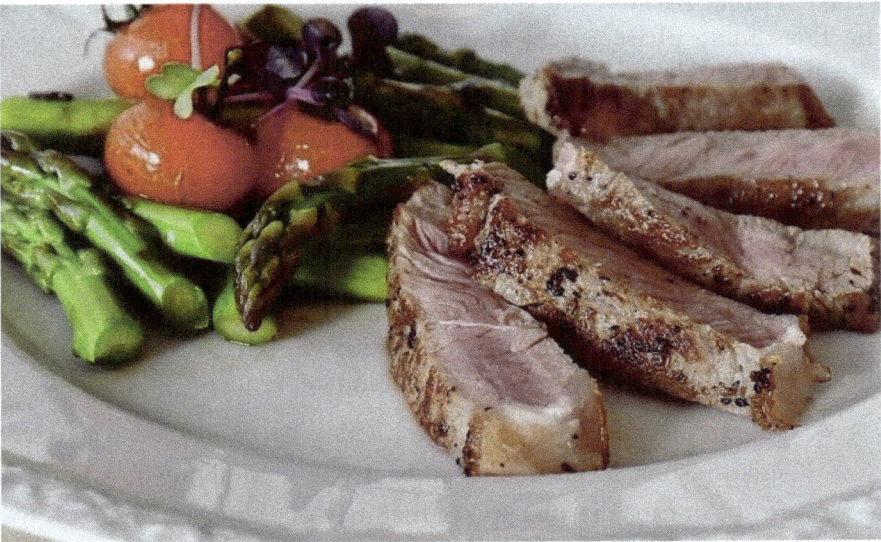

What Is the Atkins Diet?

Because it's low-carb, the Atkins diet allows for high protein and fat intake. The idea behind the Atkins diet is that by eliminating a high carb intake, the body can use the stored, excess fat as fuel. By using stored fat for energy, the body supposedly receives a consistent flow of energy and maintains the same energy levels throughout the day.

The Atkins diet contains four phases outlined below:

Phase One: This is the induction phase. Limit your carb intake to just 20 grams a day for two weeks. A majority of your meals will consist of high-fat, high protein items served with low-carb vegetables like spinach or kale. It is also best to avoid fruits and high-carb vegetables like carrots, potatoes, and turnips.

Phase Two: The balancing phase. In this phase, you will add more nuts and low-carb vegetables. You will also begin to add more fruits (healthy carbs) back into your diet.

Phase Three: By now you should be close to your goal weight. This is the fine-tuning phase where weight loss begins to slow down as you introduce more healthy carbs into your diet.

Phase Four: The final phase is the maintenance phase. At this point, you should be at your goal weight. Try to incorporate as many healthy carbs as you desire throughout the day. However, You should be mindful not to regain weight due to the higher carb intake.

The key in all these phases is to include healthy carbs in your diet. After the first two weeks, there is little restriction on what you can eat, but there are a few things that you should eliminate, such as:

- Sugar: sugar is a carbohydrate; added or processed sugar will spike insulin levels significantly. Even natural sugars found in fruit can cause insulin spikes that may put you at greater risk for diabetes.
- Grains: specifically processed grains like white flour and pasta. These are high in calories, have little nutrients, and can also spike insulin levels. When adding grains to your meal plans, keep them at a very small portion and choose whole grains like quinoa and barley.

- Vegetable oils: most vegetable oils contain a high amount of omega-6 fatty acid. Consuming these fatty acids puts you at greater risk for developing heart disease, diabetes, and cardiovascular disease.
- Diet foods: most prepackaged diet foods will have hidden carbohydrates in them.
- Low-fat foods: fat consumption is encouraged to help reduce sugar cravings. Many low-fat foods contain higher amounts of sugars and additives.
- Processed foods: especially those containing hydrogenated oils, trans fats, and partially-hydrogenated ingredients.

On the Atkins diet, meals will consist of:

- red meats
- poultry
- fatty fish and seafood
- eggs
- low-carb vegetables
- full-fat dairy
- nuts
- seeds
- healthy fats (avocado, extra virgin olive oil, coconut oil)

When it comes to what to drink, you can have water, coffee, green tea, and dry wines. Try to avoid beverages with high amounts of added sugar like soda and high-carb drinks such as beer.

Benefits

There is a great deal of research that shows the benefits of this diet. If you have been wondering whether the Atkins diet is the right fit for you, the benefits you can experience outlined below may sway you to give it a try.

Effective for Weight Loss

During the first phase of this diet, you can lose up to 15 pounds. Most of this is in water weight but you should continue to lose weight in the second phase as you make better food choices and limit your carb intake. Carbohydrates make up more than half of most people's diets and are not typically nutrient-dense. By eating this way, you are simply consuming empty calories which pack on the pounds. When you cut them out, you will reduce your calorie intake which is what allows you to lose weight.

Reduces Appetite

Many studies suggest that eating more protein and fat helps suppress appetite. An article published in *Physiology and Behavior* reviewed over 50 trials showing the correlation between higher protein consumption and appetite. In short-term trials, higher protein consumption decreased hunger and ghrelin levels (Kohanmoo et al., 2020). Ghrelin is the hunger hormone; when more of it is found in the body, appetite also increases. These studies indicate that you feel full for longer periods of time because appetite is decreased when consuming protein. This decrease in appetite aids in weight loss and weight management.

Regulates Blood Sugar Levels

Carbohydrates are known to spike blood sugar. A diet high in carbs leads to struggles with an imbalance in glucose levels. Cutting back on carbs and eliminating refined carbohydrates from one's diet has been shown to regulate blood sugar levels. This reduces your risk of diabetes and helps with weight management.

Keeps Cholesterol Levels in Check

Low-carb diets have been shown to provide a temporary improvement in bad cholesterol by lowering triglyceride levels. Keep in mind, these studies have only shown the short-term effects on cholesterol. Long-term studies show that sticking to a high-fat, high-protein diet can cause complications which put you at greater risk for heart disease and cardiovascular disease.

Eat Fewer Calories Without Having to Count Them

The Atkins diet does not require you to count calories. When you limit the amount of carbohydrates you eat, you naturally cut back on the calories you consume. As mentioned earlier, a majority of our calories come from carbohydrates. Cutting back on carbs decreases the number of calories consumed. Not having to count calories makes losing weight easier, which is why many people like this approach. They get to enjoy eating foods that make them feel full without worrying about empty calories.

Cons

The induction phase can be hard to stick with, even though it is only two weeks. Having to stick to a restrictive diet plan for any length of time is a challenge for anyone. It is more likely that you will binge, struggle with cravings, and feel deprived during these two weeks. After the induction phase, some people are more inclined to return to old eating habits such as processed foods and refined carbohydrates. Doing this leads to greater weight gain, which in the long run, makes it even harder to lose again.

While you can add high-carb foods back into your diet to maintain your goal weight, you may need to continue indefinitely with a low-carb diet. Everybody is different. While some people can add foods containing higher carbs back into their diet without seeing a leap in weight gain, others may experience significant weight gain when adding carbs back into their diet. If you are the latter and experience weight gain from the carbs you reintroduce, you may want to consider making it a habit to exclude high-carb foods from your diet.

Studies that promote the benefits of the Atkins diet do not focus on long-term. Most studies—while favorable—only followed participants for a year or less. If you are looking for a temporary fix to your health and weight struggles, this is ideal for you. To experience the long-term benefits from these dietary changes, you may want to consider another diet to maintain and continue to improve health.

Another drawback to be aware of is that many people go overboard with high-fat foods. While things like bacon and burgers are allowed on the Atkins diet, these are not foods you would want to eat every day. Many people choose to eat processed meat which is considered low-carb and high fat, but eating these in excess can put you at greater risk for other health conditions.

Weight loss can slow down significantly after the first week or two, which can be discouraging. This is true with any diet requiring substantial changes to what you eat. During the first week of phase one, you are initiating weight loss. Many people will see the number on the scale drop significantly because most of the weight they are losing is water weight. This loss is due to a higher intake of fat and the body switching from its preferred fuel source (carbohydrates) to stored fat. After your initial weight loss, you may notice that the scale barely moves. This is not to say the diet isn't working, but the first week can give many people a false sense of easy and fast weight loss.

To keep this diet low-carb, it's common to completely cut out food groups like fruit and nutrient-dense vegetables. This puts you at a higher risk for nutrient deficiencies and can lead to electrolyte imbalances.

Getting Started

The Atkins diet is pretty flexible. After the first two weeks, you will slowly begin to add healthy carbs and low-carb vegetables back into your routine. Only during this induction phase are there major restrictions on the foods you eat.

A typical meal will include a healthy serving of protein, healthy fat, and vegetables. A helpful tip to stick with the Atkins diet is to start by adding in low-carb vegetables instead of bread, pasta, rice, or potatoes. You can do this by cooking half the amount of pasta that you would typically make. To make up for that, you can add vegetables like zucchini or broccoli—both which are high in fiber.

Create your meals around protein. This should be the star of your meals. Be sure to use lean cuts of meat to get the most benefits out of it.

Having healthy snacks in between meals such as hard-boiled eggs, cheese, and nuts are allowed. Fresh fruit can also be a great snack option after the induction phase. This will allow you to curb hunger pangs and cravings without having to choose something convenient, which will often be full of carbs and sugar.

A way to combat this is to plan your meals and grocery lists. When you are getting started on any diet you will have greater success if you plan everything out ahead of time. Having a list of what you are buying from the store will reduce the risk of filling your cart with items that you do not need. Planning your meals will eliminate having to create new ideas as the week goes by, which is essential for those who have busy schedules. If you know you constantly go for quick and easy meals, prepping ahead of time will give you the same luxury but will result in healthier options.

Even after you have reached your goal weight, it is best to stick with lower-carb foods to reduce the risk of quickly gaining the weight back. Remember, you want to adopt eating habits you can stick with long-term. If you want to keep the weight off, you should use this diet as a lifestyle choice not just a weight loss solution.

7-Day Meal Plan (For Induction Phase)

Monday

Breakfast: Hard-boiled eggs and spinach topped with avocado.

Lunch: Tuna salad (made with full-fat mayo).

Dinner: Steak, roasted broccoli, and garlic, drizzled with melted grass-fed butter.

Tuesday

Breakfast: Two strips of turkey bacon and two eggs cooked any way you like.

Lunch: Chicken salad (made with full-fat mayo) over leafy greens, topped with cheddar cheese and Caesar dressing.

Dinner: Bunless cheeseburger served with a cup of cooked vegetables such as asparagus, brussel sprouts, yellow squash, or zucchini.

Wednesday

Breakfast: Spinach omelet topped with cheddar cheese.

Lunch: Roasted asparagus over leafy greens with walnuts and balsamic vinaigrette. If using store-bought dressing, check that it has no more than three grams of carbs per serving, and only use three tablespoons.

Dinner: Baked chicken breast, buffalo-style cauliflower, and leafy greens topped with cheddar cheese and extra virgin olive oil.

Thursday

Breakfast: Protein Smoothie (1 scoop Atkins approved protein powder, 1 cup spinach, ½ cup avocado, ice for desired thickness).

Lunch: Egg salad over leafy greens topped with bacon bits, cheddar cheese, and extra virgin olive oil.

Dinner: Grilled pork chops with zucchini and summer squash sautéed in grass-fed butter.

Friday

Breakfast: Mushroom and cheddar omelet.

Lunch: Chicken salad over leafy greens.

Dinner: Sautéed beef strips with onions and asparagus (cooked with grass-fed butter).

Saturday

Breakfast: Four strips of bacon and two eggs cooked any way, plus one cup of sautéed spinach (cooked with grass-fed butter).

Lunch: Smoothie (1 ½ cups almond milk, 1 scoop Atkins approved protein powder, 1 cup spinach, ½ cup avocado, ice for desired thickness).

Dinner: Pork kabobs with onion, bell pepper, and zucchini.

Sunday

Breakfast: Chorizo, eggs, and spinach skillet.

Lunch: Goat cheese salad with spinach, olives, cherry tomatoes, cucumber, and extra virgin olive oil.

Dinner: Chef salad with chicken.

Snack ideas for Phase 1:
- celery with cream cheese
- hard-boiled eggs
- sliced ham or turkey rolled with cheddar cheese
- string cheese
- raw vegetables (bell pepper, celery sticks, cucumbers)
- cucumber with tuna salad
- olives

- cheddar cheese lettuce wraps

7-Day Meal Plan (After Induction Phase)

Monday

Breakfast: Two eggs with a small serving of fruit.

Lunch: Salad with tomato, cucumber, onion, and cheese, drizzled with olive oil and balsamic vinegar.

Dinner: Pulled pork with cauliflower mash.

Tuesday

Breakfast: Nut Butter and Strawberry Smoothie (two cups spinach or kale, four frozen strawberries, one teaspoon chia seeds, two tablespoons almond butter, one cup almond milk, and one tablespoon maple syrup or honey).

Lunch: Bell peppers stuffed with tuna salad.

Dinner: Grilled chicken breast with zucchini noodles and alfredo sauce.

Wednesday

Breakfast: Two fried eggs and two sausage links.

Lunch: Ham, turkey, cheese, and hard-boiled eggs served over leafy greens topped with ranch.

Dinner: Chicken stir fry with cauliflower rice, peppers, onions, mushrooms, and broccoli.

Thursday

Breakfast: Full-fat yogurt topped with fresh fruit and granola.

Lunch: Apple, tuna, and celery salad served over leafy greens.

Dinner: Stuffed bell peppers (stuff with cauliflower rice, beef, onions, and mushrooms).

Friday

Breakfast: Veggie omelet with cheese.

Lunch: Grilled chicken breast with roasted broccoli and red peppers.

Dinner: Shrimp Cobb salad with dijon mustard dressing.

Saturday

Breakfast: Two eggs, ham, and cheese served with sautéed spinach.

Lunch: Baked chicken with tomatoes, spinach, and cheese topped with extra virgin olive oil and balsamic vinaigrette.

Dinner: Grilled pork tenderloin with puréed cauliflower and steamed vegetables.

Sunday

Breakfast: Nut Butter and Strawberry Smoothie (two cups spinach or kale, four frozen strawberries, one teaspoon chia seeds, two tablespoons almond butter, one cup almond milk, and one tablespoon maple syrup or honey).

Lunch: Chicken and avocado salad served over spinach topped with fresh lime juice and cilantro.

Dinner: Grilled salmon with green beans and asparagus.

Snacks for Phases 2-4:

- all snacks from phase one
- fresh fruit: melon, strawberries, and blueberries
- celery with nut butter
- nuts
- seeds
- cottage cheese
- yogurt topped with coconut

Chapter 2:

DASH Diet

The DASH diet stands for dietary approach to stop hypertension and was designed by individuals of The National Heart, Blood, and Lung Institute to help people lower blood pressure. The DASH diet is considered a low-sodium and low-salt diet but emphasizes nutrient-rich foods. If you want a diet plan that has simple guidelines with few restrictions, the DASH diet might be for you.

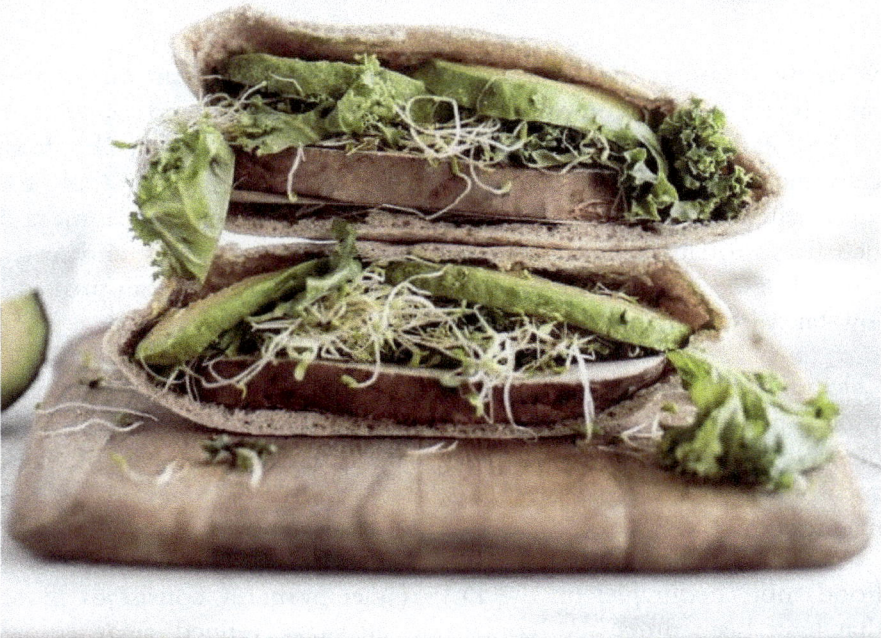

What Is the DASH Diet?

This is a heart-healthy eating plan which focuses on a balanced diet. There are no strict requirements; instead, the diet outlines nutritional goals you can use as a guide for planning meals during the week.

Based on a 2,000 calorie diet, the following servings are suggested:

- Grains: six to eight servings a day.
- Red meat, poultry, and fish: six or less servings a day.
- Vegetables: four to five servings a day.
- Fruit: four to five servings a day.
- Low-fat or fat-free dairy: two to three servings a day.
- Fats and oils: two to three servings a day.
- Sodium: no more than 2,300 mg a day.
- Beans, nuts, seeds, and peas: four to five servings a day.
- Sweets: less than five servings a day.

While there are no hard-cut restrictions on what you can eat on this diet, there are recommendations. Carbohydrates should consist of healthy starches which include leafy green vegetables, fruit with a low-glycemic index, whole grains, and legumes or beans. Opt for unsaturated fats like avocado, olive oil, nuts, flax seeds, and omega-3 rich fish. Proteins should be plant-based like legumes, nuts, and seeds. Animal-based proteins are fine as well but try to stick to lean proteins, low-fat dairy, and eggs.

Calcium, potassium, and magnesium-rich foods are highly encouraged while on the DASH diet. Dairy and green, leafy vegetables provide plenty of calcium. Foods rich in potassium include bananas, oranges, and spinach. Leafy vegetables, nuts, seeds, and whole grains are rich in magnesium.

Foods not encouraged on the DASH diet primarily consist of those that have been processed, contain added sugar, refined sugar, or are high in sodium.

Benefits

Although the DASH diet is designed to combat high blood pressure, it can also lead to making food choices that will help you lose and maintain a healthy weight. There are additional benefits you will experience when you lower your blood pressure and if you are at greater risk for high blood pressure, carefully consider transitioning to this type of diet.

Lowers Blood Pressure

The DASH diet puts an emphasis on restricting sodium intake. Numerous studies show that cutting down on sodium can result in significantly lower blood pressure levels. One such study published by the U.S. Department of Health and Human Services had 412 participants. Half of the participants followed the DASH diet plan, while the other half stuck with a typical Western diet. For the first month, both groups consumed 3,330 milligrams of sodium a day, the second month consumed 2,300 milligrams of sodium, and the third month consumed 1,500 milligrams of sodium. After those three months, both groups showed a reduction in blood pressure that lowered even more when sodium intake was lower. Those in the DASH diet group saw significantly lower blood pressure levels than those following the Western diet plan (Juraschek et al., 2020). The studies proved that lower sodium intake—despite eating habits—will help lower blood pressure but those who follow a nutrient-dense diet, like the DASH diet, will benefit even more.

Reduce the Risk of Depression

A large study that included over 950 participants showed that individuals who stuck to a DASH diet were less likely to suffer from depression or symptoms of depression (Roan, 2018). Though the study does not indicate why the DASH diet impacts mood, it does highlight that the foods we consume can have an impact on our mental health just as much as our physical health.

Reduces the Risk of Heart Disease and Heart Failure

A long-term study shows that individuals who followed the DASH diet had a 40% lower risk of heart failure than those who followed any other type of diet. This study tracked individuals with an average age of 75, suggesting that older adults can benefit greatly from the DASH diet to prevent heart failure and other heart diseases without the need for medicine. An early study of participants with an average age of 45 also showed a much lower risk for heart disease (Paddock, 2019).

Helps Treat Metabolic Syndrome

Metabolic syndrome is not just one condition but a combination of multiple serious conditions that can increase the risk of heart disease, type 2 diabetes, and stroke. Some conditions include high blood pressure, insulin resistance, high blood sugar, abnormal cholesterol levels, and excess fat around the waist. When a person has more than one of these conditions, they significantly increase their chances of experiencing serious health conditions. The DASH diet has been shown to help reduce the risk of many of these conditions. When the DASH diet is combined with additional treatments to help manage metabolic syndrome, individuals will see long-term improvements in their health.

Helps Manage and Reduces the Risk of Diabetes

Those at risk of type 2 diabetes will significantly reduce their risk of developing the condition if they follow the DASH diet. The American Dietetic Association recommends that patients at risk of diabetes should:

- lower their saturated fat intake to no more than seven percent of their calorie intake.

- reduce or eliminate consumption of trans fats
- reduce their cholesterol to 200 milligrams a day or lower.
- reduce added sugar consumption, especially sugar from beverages.

The DASH diet helps individuals meet all the above recommendations (Challa et al., 2021).

Cons

A common complaint from those who switch from a Western diet to the DASH diet is digestive discomfort. These issues occur when you drastically consume more fiber-rich foods like fruits and vegetables. This can be easily avoided by slowly increasing your intake of high-fiber foods and increasing your water intake at the same time.

Some may struggle to transition to this diet because of having to limit their salt intake. Most Americans consume well over 3,400 mg of sodium a day (Frey, 2020). Skimping on the salt can be a hard habit for some to break. The DASH diet recommends cutting down to 2,300 mg and eventually 1500 mg a day. Additionally, the lower sodium intake takes more work when prepping meals. With many other diets, there is some flexibility when incorporating prepackaged, healthy meals. These meals often have higher sodium levels so you may have to bypass them on the DASH diet and stick with preparing and making your own meals instead.

While it is not required for you to keep track of calories, you need to be meticulous about the servings of each food group you consume throughout the day. Since these servings are based on caloric intake, you should do some calorie counting to ensure you are getting the right balance of each food group. This can be tedious and overwhelming for those who want a straightforward and simple approach to weight loss.

Weight loss on the DASH diet is slow-moving. The diet was not initially designed for weight loss but instead, for many other health benefits which can help maintain a healthy weight. Making dietary changes like limiting sugar intake and choosing to eat more vegetables can lead to weight loss, just do not expect a quick slim down or even a fast track weight loss plan on the DASH diet.

You may also experience a change in your taste buds. Eliminating salt and excess sugar from foods is bound to make them taste differently. Some do not like the way their taste preferences change. You need to give your palate some time to adjust to your new way of eating just as your body needs time to adjust. After a while, you may notice that you enjoy your food more than you used to because you get the true flavors of your foods coming through.

The DASH diet is not for everyone; those with certain health conditions such as kidney or liver disease may want to reconsider this diet. Individuals who have these conditions may find their condition worsens by sticking to the DASH diet. Other conditions that will require modification to the DASH diet include:

- Individuals with chronic heart failure.
- Those who have type 2 diabetes and do not have a treatment plan to help manage those symptoms.
- Individuals who are lactose intolerant
- Individuals who have been diagnosed with celiac disease or who have a gluten intolerance.

If you have an underlying medical condition, it is best to consult with your physician to understand your risk and options. It is also a wise choice to work with a dietitian or nutritionist to ensure you are making the right choice in managing your conditions and nutrition.

Getting Started

When deciding on which foods to eat on the DASH diet, consider the following: It is important to choose foods that will help you control blood pressure levels. To accomplish this, keep the following in mind:

- Choose foods low in saturated fats.
- Go with foods high in calcium, potassium, magnesium, and fiber.
- Choose foods high in protein.
- When possible, opt for low sodium foods.
- Avoid overeating fatty meats, full-fat dairy, sweetened beverages, candy, desserts, and excess sodium.
- For optimal weight loss, limit your intake of starchy vegetables like potatoes, corn, and winter squash.

7-Day Meal Plan

Monday

Breakfast: 2 boiled eggs, 2 slices of turkey bacon, ½ cup cherry tomatoes, and ½ cup of black beans with 2 slices of whole-wheat toast.

Snack: A banana.

Lunch: Grilled tuna salad with 2 cups of leafy greens, ½ cup cherry tomatoes, and 2 tablespoons low-fat dressing.

Snack: ½ cup of pears and 1 cup of low-fat yogurt.

Dinner: Whole wheat spaghetti with meatballs and a side of green peas.

Tuesday

Breakfast: Two slices of whole-wheat toast with two tablespoons of nut butter and a banana.

Snack: An apple.

Lunch: 3-ounces of grilled chicken, 1 cup roasted vegetables, and 1 cup of brown rice topped with 1 ½ ounces of low-fat cheese.

Snack: A cup of fruit salad.

Dinner: A 3-ounce steak, 1 cup of roasted vegetables, and ½ cup of lentils.

Wednesday

Breakfast: 1 cup of oats with 1 cup of low-fat milk and ½ cup of blueberries.

Snack: An orange.

Lunch: Grilled tuna salad with 1 boiled egg, 2 cups of leafy greens, ½ cup cherry tomatoes, and 2 tablespoons of low-fat dressing.

Snack: 4 whole grain crackers, ½ cup pineapple chunks, and 1 ½ ounces of low-fat cottage cheese.

Dinner: A 3-ounce chicken breast with ½ cup steamed broccoli and ½ cup steam carrots. Serve with 1 cup of brown rice.

Thursday

Breakfast: Green Smoothie (1 banana, 1 cup spinach, ½ cup fat-free milk, ¼ cup oats, ¾ cup frozen mango, and ¼ cup nonfat yogurt).

Snack: An apple.

Lunch: 2 slices of whole-wheat bread with 3 ounces of lean turkey topped with low-fat cheese, ½ cup of green salad with ½ cup of cherry tomatoes and 2 tablespoons of low-fat dressing.

Snack: Fruit salad and a cup of low-fat yogurt.

Dinner: A 3-ounce salmon with 1 cup of boiled potatoes and 1 ½ cups boiled vegetables.

Friday

Breakfast: 1 cup of oats topped with cinnamon.

Snack: 1 cup yogurt.

Lunch: 3 ounces of chicken salad over 2 cups of leafy greens, ½ cup of cherry tomatoes, ½ teaspoon of sunflower seeds, and 4 whole-grain crackers.

Snack: 1 banana and ½ cup of almonds.

Dinner: Beef kabobs made with 3 ounces of beef, 1 cup of peppers, onions, mushrooms, and cherry tomatoes. Served with a cup of wild rice.

Saturday

Breakfast: 1 bran muffin and 1 cup of fresh fruit topped with a ⅓ cup of walnuts and 1 cup of fat-free yogurt.

Snack: An orange.

Lunch: Chicken wrap (3 ounces of chicken, ½ tablespoon mayo, and ½ cup spinach, wrapped in a whole-wheat tortilla) with a side of ½ cup of baby carrots.

Snack: Trail mix (¼ cup raisins, about 15 unsalted, mini twist pretzels, and 1 tablespoon of sunflower seeds).

Dinner: Cauliflower steak with sautéed spinach, roasted carrots, and green peas.

Sunday

Breakfast: A slice of whole-wheat bread topped with an egg (cooked in olive oil) and two tablespoons of salsa with one banana.

Snack: Banana Smoothie (two bananas, a tablespoon of honey, a cup of nonfat milk, and a cup of nonfat yogurt).

Lunch: White bean avocado salad (2 cups of leafy greens, ¼ cup cucumber, ¼ cup cherry tomatoes, ¼ cup celery, ⅓ cup white beans, and ½ an avocado, topped with two tablespoons of vinaigrette).

Snack: An apple and one cup of low-fat yogurt

Dinner: Chicken chili with sweet potatoes. Top with avocado slices and nonfat plain Greek yogurt.

Chapter 3:

Detox and Cleansing Diets

A detox or cleanse is designed to give you a clean slate when starting a new healthy diet. There have been plenty of fad detox and cleanse diets from the grapefruit detox to the fruit juice cleanse; some are shown to be effective while others can have terrible side effects. There are also plenty of products that market themselves as a magical solution for weight loss. Understand that while some detox and cleansing diets can help you drop pounds, many of them can be a disappointment. Doing a cleanse can significantly reduce bloating, help you feel more energized, and can be a great way to jumpstart your weight loss journey.

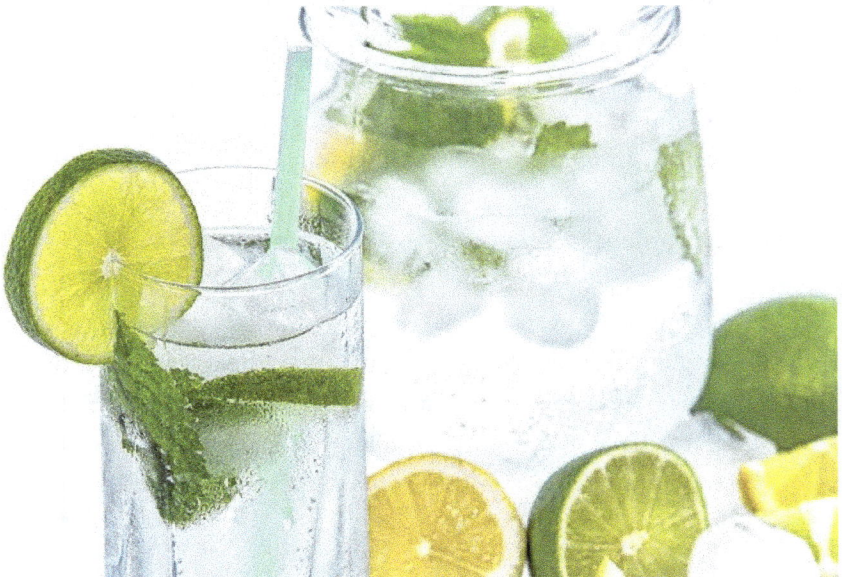

What Is a Detox and Cleansing Diet?

A detox and cleansing diet is a diet that focuses on eliminating toxins from the body while cleansing specific areas such as the colon, the liver, or the blood. Diets of this kind require a short fasting period followed by a period of strict diet limitations. It is common for individuals to drink their nutrients, such as only drinking herbal teas, juices, or water. Other detoxes may involve more specific cleanses, such as a colon cleanse or enema.

There are a variety of ways to complete a detox diet. Most diets in this category require one or more of the following:

- A one to three-day fast.
- Only drink fresh fruit or vegetable juices, smoothies, tea, or water.
- Only drink salted water or lemon water. Salt water triggers the body's natural detox process. It also helps the digestive tract remove waste build-up. Lemon water will help flush toxins from the body. It also provides you with vitamin C which helps restore the liver so it can function better.
- Eliminate all foods that contain high amounts of heavy metals, contaminants, and allergens. Fish is the most common food containing heavy metals, but many fruits and vegetables can also have metals in them depending on the soil where they are grown.
- Incorporate supplements and herbs into your daily routine.
- Remove all allergenic foods for five days, then slowly reintroduce these foods one at a time. Removing common allergens like dairy, nuts, eggs, and wheat can give the body time to heal from the damage these foods cause. Even if you do not have a known food allergy it can still be a good idea to temporarily remove these foods to recognize any possible discomforts.
- Exercise daily.
- Eliminate alcohol, coffee, and refined sugar from your diet.
- Quit smoking.

There are many programs available that provide you with the necessary steps and products to consume while doing a cleanse. It is a better idea to avoid participating in a cleansing program or purchasing a cleansing kit. Many of these products are not considered safe and few studies have been conducted on the safety of partaking in the program. This goes for detox supplements and cleansing tea products. Many herbal supplements and detox teas contain laxatives. This is done to give you the impression that these capsules and drinks are doing their job but they really don't do anything to help with weight loss or health.

A more natural approach to detoxing the body and jumpstart your weight loss journey is to try a short three-day cleanse that includes one or more of the following detox drinks:

- Lemon and Ginger Detox: Ginger helps aid in digestion and better digestion makes losing weight easier. Lemon helps stimulate the digestive tract, which is why many people recommend drinking water with fresh squeezed lemon first thing in the morning when you are trying to lose weight. Lemons also contain important antioxidants that help fight off free radicals that can wreak havoc on your body. You can create a lemon and ginger detox drink by squeezing half a lemon into an 8-ounce glass of warm water and adding an inch-long piece of fresh ginger.

- Cinnamon and Honey Detox: Cinnamon can help get rid of cravings and reduce inflammation in the body. Raw organic honey contains properties that help improve metabolism. Better metabolism helps you use the calories you consume in the most effective way. To create the cinnamon honey detox drink add a tablespoon of honey and half a tablespoon of cinnamon to an 8-ounce glass of warm water. You can drink this whenever you get a craving for something sweet or feel like you need to eat out of boredom or uncomfortable emotions.

- Cucumber and Mint Detox: Cucumbers contain a high amount of water and beneficial antioxidants. These components help fight against free radicals but also assist in flushing the system of toxins. Mint helps aid in digestion. You can create a cucumber and mint detox drink by filling a pitcher with water, adding some cucumber slices, and fresh mint leaves. Allow the mixture to infuse for about an hour then drink it throughout the day to stay hydrated and refreshed.

- Green Tea Detox: Green tea is raved about because of its antioxidants but it includes other properties that can aid in your weight loss goals. Consuming green tea can help protect against free radicals and reduce the production of these harmful chemicals. It also activates the body's natural fat-burning system which will help you drop a few pounds without any effort. Simply brew organic green tea and drink it two or three times a day.

- Cranberry Detox: Cranberry juice is a natural way to help alleviate symptoms of urinary tract infections because of its useful antioxidants. These same antioxidants can combat infections, flush the digestive tract of toxins, and may even help improve cholesterol levels. You want to ensure you choose organic cranberry juice with no added sugar. Drink this juice a few times a day to get the full benefit.

Benefits

Many people choose to do a detox cleanse to help alleviate abdominal bloat. These types of short-term diets can also help you feel more energized and refreshed. There are a few other benefits that make a detox and cleanse diet the right choice for those looking to get started with losing weight and feeling healthier.

Removes Toxins and Environmental Pollutants

A detox cleansing diet is recommended when an individual has been exposed to environmental toxins like pollutants, chemicals, or heavy metals and harmful compounds. Most of these diets work to stimulate the liver to help remove excess toxins from the body. The most common toxins eliminated through a detox diet include persistent organic pollutants (POPs), heavy metals, bisphenol A (BPA), and phthalates (Bjarnadottir, 2019). There are a few other benefits listed below that might entice you to commit to a short detox and cleanse diet.

Increase Nutrients and Proper Absorption of Nutrients

Most detox and cleanse diets emphasize eating fresh fruits and vegetables or drinking them as a natural juice. This provides the body with essential nutrients that it may have been lacking. Most detox drinks, like those mentioned previously, contain beneficial antioxidants and other compounds that can help improve health in various ways.

Jumpstart Weight Loss

Most detox and cleanse diets require calorie restrictions. Cutting back on calories will almost always lead to weight loss. It is not uncommon for individuals to lose three pounds or more after completing a detox cleanse. This can provide essential motivation to help you stick with a healthy eating plan after your detox and cleansing period.

Cons

Many who partake in a detox diet have admitted to not feeling very well during the process. Any type of fasting or extreme calorie restriction as recommended on a detox diet can leave you feeling tired and irritable.

Weight loss from a detox can occur rapidly, but the weight usually comes back on unless you have a clear diet plan to follow after the detox. It's important to note the weight you lose from a detox is not going to be fat. In most instances, the pounds you shed while doing a detox is from muscle mass or water weight. If you immediately pick up poor eating habits following a cleanse, the weight will come back plus some. When you deprive the body of food and significantly restrict calories, it goes into survival mode. The next time you eat you are bound to store a little extra because the body is confused about when food will be supplied again. Doing this too often eventually leads to incredibly stubborn body fat that will take much longer to work off.

Detoxing for any length of time can also cause additional stress hormones to be released. These stress hormones can wreak havoc on your body by causing inflammation, making it harder to sleep, and increasing your appetite.

Resisting temptation and struggling with extreme hunger makes it hard to stay committed to a detox diet. Even if it is just three days, many people will not feel as energized or in good spirits from depriving their body of actual food.

If you are doing a colon cleanse with your detox, there are more unpleasant side effects to be aware of. These cleanses can cause dehydration, so it is vital to drink plenty of liquids. You may also feel cramping, bloating, or nausea while detoxing.

There is also much debate about how effective a detox and cleansing diet is at ridding the body of toxins. The liver already does a fairly thorough job of ridding toxins from the body and while some detoxes may help aid the liver, studies have revealed conflicting results about their effectiveness.

Children, young adults, older adults, pregnant women or those who are nursing, and individuals with blood sugar conditions like diabetes should not take part in a detox or cleansing diet. It is also advised to speak to your primary care physician before considering a detox or cleansing diet.

Getting Started

First you should decide how long you will stick with your detox. Remember, this is not meant to be long-term, only three to seven days. Once you have decided on a length of time you need to consider what healthy habits you will add to your day after your cleanse. Completing a detox cleanse and returning to your old eating habits is a waste of time. This will quickly cause you to gain the weight back after putting in all that effort for nothing. Consider the lifestyle changes you want to make when it comes to food and have a plan in place to start as soon as your detox period is done.

3-Day Detox Plan

You can start a 3-day detox on any day, ensuring that you commit to the diet for three consecutive days. You will follow the same meal plan for all three days.

Days 1, 2, and 3

Breakfast: Prebiotic Smoothie (½ cup rolled oats, 1 banana, 1 teaspoon ground flax seed, 1 teaspoon raw cacao, ½ cup almond milk, and ½ cup water).

Follow the smoothie with an 8-ounce glass of warm lemon and ginger water.

Snack: Green juice (1 cup of kale, 1 cucumber, 2 celery stalks, juice from 1 lemon, and a teaspoon fresh grated ginger or a ½-inch piece).

Lunch: Green Smoothie (1 ½ cups of almond milk, ¼ avocado, 1 tablespoon pure vanilla extract, and 1 teaspoon of cinnamon).

Dinner: Large mixed green salad with roasted vegetables, topped with fresh lemon juice and avocado, and a baked sweet potato on the side.

7-Day Detox Plan

Monday

Breakfast: Green Juice (½ an avocado. ¼ cup coconut milk, ½ cup almond milk, 1 teaspoon fresh grated ginger, ½ teaspoon turmeric, juice from ½ a lime, and 1 teaspoon pure maple syrup if desired).

Snack: Green Tea

Lunch: A cup of raw celery, cucumbers, bell peppers, or carrots (or a combination of two or more).

Snack: Fresh squeezed juice (one carrot, a beet, an apple, one cucumber, and a celery stalk).

Dinner: Mixed green salad and half an avocado topped with fresh lemon juice.

Tuesday

Breakfast: Prebiotic Smoothie (blend together ½ cup rolled oats, 1 banana, a teaspoon ground flax seed, a teaspoon raw cacao, ½ cup almond milk, and ½ cup of water).

Follow the smoothie with a tall glass of warm water with lemon.

Snack: Green tea.

Lunch: A cup of raw celery, cucumbers, bell peppers, or carrots (or a combination of two or more).

Snack: Fresh squeezed juice (blend together segments of 1 red grapefruit, 2 cups pineapple chunks, 1 teaspoon fresh grated ginger, ¼ cup of water, and ¼ cup fresh mint leaves).

Dinner: Large mixed green salad with roasted vegetables topped with fresh lemon juice and a baked sweet potato on the side.

Wednesday

Breakfast: Coconut Pineapple Smoothie (1 ½ cups of coconut water, 2 cups of kale, ¼ of an avocado, and ½ cup of pineapple).

Snack: Green tea.

Lunch: A cup of raw celery, cucumbers, bell peppers, or carrots (or a combination of two or more).

Snack: Fresh squeezed juice (one carrot, two oranges, half an inch piece of raw turmeric, half an inch piece of ginger, and juice from half a lemon).

Dinner: Kale salad (remove the ribs from a large bunch of kale and massage the leaves with lemon juice until they begin to wilt). Top with a quarter of an avocado and raw vegetables.

Thursday

Breakfast: Prebiotic Smoothie (½ cup rolled oats, 1 banana, 1 teaspoon ground flax seed, 1 teaspoon raw cacao, ½ cup almond milk, and ½ cup of water).

After the smoothie, drink a large glass of warm water with lemon.

Snack: Green Tea

Lunch: A cup of raw celery, cucumbers, bell peppers, or carrots (or a combination of two or more).

Snack: Fresh squeezed juice (1 fresh aloe vera leaf, ½ cup chopped beetroot, 2 cups pomegranate juice, ¼ teaspoon black pepper powder).

Dinner: Mixed green salad and half an avocado topped with fresh lemon juice.

Friday

Breakfast: Avocado Smoothie (1 ½ cups of almond milk, ½ cup of frozen cherries, 2 cups of kale, ½ an avocado, 2 teaspoons of pure vanilla extract, and 1 teaspoon of cinnamon).

Snack: Green tea.

Lunch: A cup of raw celery, cucumbers, bell peppers, or carrots (or a combination of two or more).

Snack: Fresh squeezed juice (one carrot, a beet, an apple, one cucumber, and a celery stalk).

Dinner: Mixed green salad and half an avocado topped with fresh lemon juice and a baked sweet potato.

Saturday

Breakfast: Green juice (a cup of kale, a cucumber, two celery stalks, juice from one lemon, and a teaspoon of fresh grated ginger or a half-inch piece).

Snack: Green tea.

Lunch: A cup of raw celery, cucumbers, bell peppers, or carrots (or a combination of two or more).

Snack: Smoothie (blend together a cup of almond milk, four celery stalks, a cucumber, a cup of kale, half a green apple, half a lime, a cup of pineapple, and a tablespoon of coconut oil).

Dinner: Mixed green salad and half an avocado topped with fresh lemon juice.

Sunday

Breakfast: Detox drink (2 tablespoon apple cider vinegar, 2 tablespoons fresh lemon juice, ½ teaspoon fresh ground ginger, ¼ teaspoon cinnamon, ¼ teaspoon cayenne pepper, and 1 teaspoon raw organic honey). If you find the taste of the apple cider vinegar too overbearing, follow it with a small amount of warm water.

Snack: Green tea.

Lunch: A cup of raw celery, cucumbers, bell peppers, or carrots (or a combination of two or more).

Snack: Green Smoothie (1 ½ cups of almond milk, ¼ avocado, 1 tablespoon pure vanilla extract, and 1 teaspoon of cinnamon).

Dinner: Kale salad (remove the ribs from a large bunch of kale and massage the leaves with lemon juice until they begin to wilt). Top with ¼ of an avocado and raw vegetables.

Chapter 4:

Flexitarian Diet

The flexitarian diet is a flexible vegetarian diet. While the diet's main focus is to eat primarily plant-based foods, there is no elimination of animal products or meat. This gives people the benefits of eating vegetarian food with the option to enjoy a burger or steak every once in a while. This diet is favored by those who want to eat more fruits and vegetables but do not want to completely cut out some of their favorite foods. Read on to learn if a flexitarian diet is the right diet for you and your health goals.

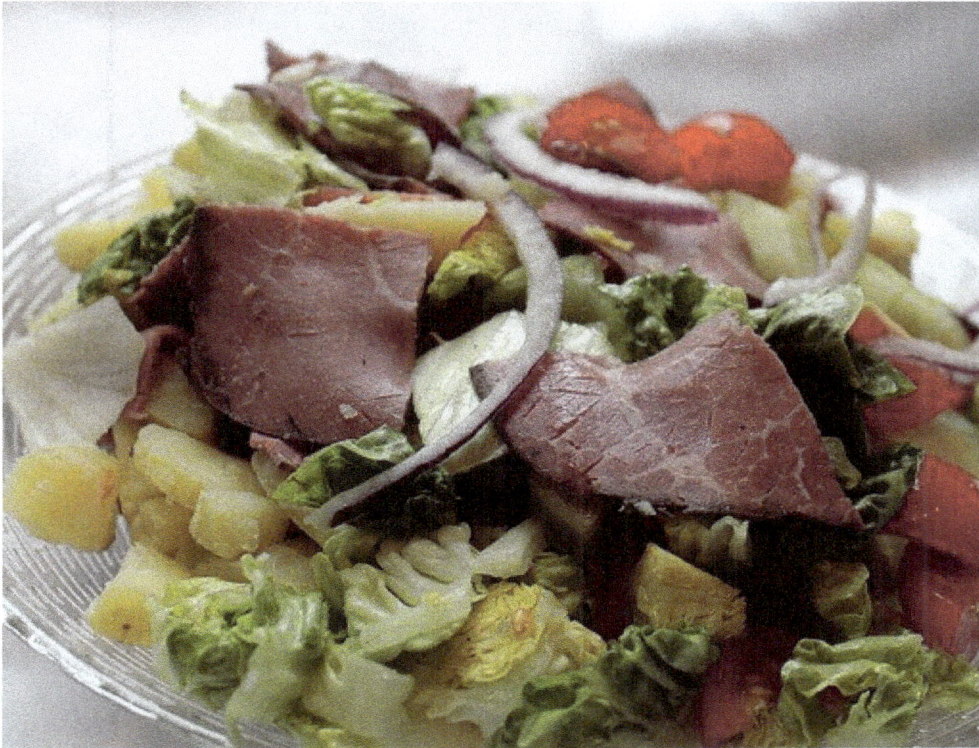

What Is the Flexitarian Diet?

Unlike full-on vegetarianism, animal products and meats are not forbidden or compelled to be eliminated. Instead, this diet encourages you to slowly decrease your consumption of these items and enjoy them sparingly. Below, you will find a food list to use as a guide for the best foods to eat on the flexitarian diet:

- plant proteins
- whole grains
- vegetables
- fruits
- nuts and nut butter
- seeds
- tofu
- healthy fats (avocados, extra virgin olive oil)
- plant or dairy milk

Foods that are suggested to cut back on include:

- red meat and animal proteins
- poultry
- seafood
- animal fats (butter, cream, whole milk)
- processed refined grains (white pasta, white bread, white rice)
- processed foods (pastries and chips)
- high sugar beverages (soda, fruit juices)

For those who like to count calories or who need to have a more structured outline for their meal plans can refer to the following breakdown:

- Breakfast should be around 300 calories
- Lunch should be around 400 calories
- Dinner should be around 500 calories

- Snacks should be no more than 150 calories. Incorporate two snacks a day.

This plan equals 15oo calories a day which can be easily adjusted if you need to reduce your calorie intake to help you lose weight or increase calories to help maintain a healthy weight.

Benefits

There are many reasons people lean toward a flexitarian diet. It is easy to transition to and can make switching to a more plant-based diet feasible. The simplified guidelines can jumpstart weight loss but there are many reasons you might want to consider going with a flexitarian diet.

Helps Reduce the Risk of Diabetes

Various studies have been conducted that show non-vegetarians have a significantly higher risk of developing diabetes. In one study, individuals who consumed a vegetarian diet were 25% less likely to develop metabolic syndrome which is often a precursor to type 2 diabetes (Derbyshire, 2017).

Easy to Follow and Maintain

The flexitarian diet does not require you to count calories or completely eliminate foods from your diet. You decide how often you want to eat meat and other animal products; the more you cut back the more beneficial the diet is. Because of its flexibility, the flexitarian diet can be maintained long-term.

Lose Weight and Keep It Off

A flexitarian diet focuses on eating more whole and plant-based foods. When you begin to cut out processed foods from your diet and start to fuel your body with the right nutrients, you are going to experience weight loss. Making this diet a lifestyle change can help keep weight off long-term. A study published in the *Clinic of Nutrition Research* showed that women who stuck with a semi-vegetarian diet—like the flexitarian diet—not only lost more weight but had a lower body mass index and over all body fat than those who ate a non-vegetarian diet (Kim and Bae, 2015).

Following this diet will allow you to feel fuller and consume fewer calories which will boost weight loss efforts. A flexitarian diet is packed with fiber-rich foods. Fiber makes us feel full faster when we are eating and it keeps us feeling full for longer. Many vegetables like broccoli, carrots, leafy greens, and zucchini are high in fiber and low in calories. These foods allow you to eat until you are full without adding calories. Lower caloric intake is the key to losing weight.

Lowers Risk of Heart Disease and Stroke

A diet that encourages eating more fruits and vegetables is beneficial to the heart. Eating more plant-based proteins helps lower bad cholesterol levels and can reduce your risk of heart disease.

Live Longer

Flexitarians live over three years longer than individuals who eat a primarily carnivorous diet. Various studies prove that reducing your meat intake can help increase longevity. When you eliminate most animal products from your diet and rely on plant-based sources, you increase the nutrients your body receives. These extra nutrients not only help reduce the risk of various health conditions but allow the body to function optimally for many years.

Cons

Some people mistakenly approach the flexitarian diet as simply eating less meat while allowing themselves to gorge on other foods that lack nutrients. If you eat pastries and pasta with an occasional chicken breast, you will not reap the benefits of this diet.

There is also a risk of not getting the right balance of nutrients like iron, omega-3, calcium, and vitamin B12. We obtain a variety of these nutrients from animal products and if not carefully planned out, you can end up having deficiencies.

Other research suggests that a flexitarian diet can lead to more disordered eating patterns. Some people are more likely to binge or overeat on this type of flexible diet. If you are someone who needs more restrictions and specific guidelines for healthy eating, this may not be the ideal diet for you. Going fully vegetarian or vegan which completely eliminates animal products from the diet may be a better alternative than the flexitarian plan—providing the same health benefits.

Getting Started

When switching to a flexitarian diet, you want to increase your fresh fruit and vegetable consumption. Try to progressively decrease your consumption of meat; an easy approach to this would be to choose 1 or two 2 to go completely meatless. Keep your meat consumption on the other days around 26 ounces total. Once you have maintained 2 meatless days a week for 4 weeks, cut up your meatless days to 4 days a week. Keep your meat consumption on the remaining days around 18 ounces. Finally, go meatless 5 days a week and only consume around 9 ounces of meat on the remaining days. This still allows you to have a nice portion of meat on both days.

Some other helpful tips to get you started include:

- Use lots of spices and herbs to change up the flavors.
- Try one new vegetarian recipe a week.

- Make the vegetables the star of your meals. Instead of a ribeye, go with a cauliflower steak. Use meats and animal products as a side to go along with your vegetables. When you make up a plate for your meals, ensure at least half of it consists of fruits and vegetables.
- Start with a meatless breakfast. Oatmeal, smoothies, and veggie wraps are easy substitutes for eggs and bacon. This will also set you up for more success with meatless meals throughout the rest of your day.
- Add exercise to maximize your weight loss efforts. You should aim to incorporate 30 minutes of moderate exercise at least 5 days a week and 2 days of strength training at least 2 times a week. You can also increase the intensity of your workouts. With a high intensity sessions you can cut your time to just 20 minutes a day 3 days a week. Keep the 2 days of strength training, though.

7-Day Meal Plan (Two Meatless Days)

Monday (meatless)

Breakfast: Strawberry Pineapple Smoothie (blend together ¾ cup of almond milk, ½ cup of strawberries, ½ cup of pineapple, 1 cup of kale or spinach, and 1 tablespoon almond butter).

Snack: A cup of Greek Yogurt with blueberries.

Lunch: An apple with Greek salad (cucumber, tomatoes, onions, olives, and feta cheese) drizzled with extra virgin olive oil and balsamic vinegar.

Snack: Avocado toast.

Dinner: Roasted chickpeas and vegetables with leafy greens and a baked sweet potato.

Tuesday

Breakfast: Black bean, bell pepper, and pepper jack cheese omelet with a banana.

Snack: Apple slices and a tablespoon of nut butter.

Lunch: Chicken salad over mixed greens and ½ cup of melon.

Snack: Raw vegetables with hummus.

Dinner: Tofu pad thai.

Wednesday

Breakfast: Oats (made with almond milk) topped with walnuts and fresh fruit.

Snack: ½ cup of strawberries and a banana.

Lunch: Lentil soup.

Snack: A pear and ¼ cup of walnuts.

Dinner: Baked salmon, sautéed spinach, and brown rice.

Thursday

Breakfast: Black bean and egg burritos with tomatoes and avocado.

Snack: Tropical Smoothie (blend together ½ cup of almond milk, ½ cup of strawberries, ½ cup of pineapples, 1 cup of kale or spinach, and ½ tablespoon nut butter).

Lunch: Spicy buffalo cauliflower bowls topped with avocado and a green Tahini dressing.

Snack: Celery sticks with nut butter.

Dinner: Roasted chicken breast and vegetables with zucchini noodles and cashew alfredo sauce.

Friday

Breakfast: Green Smoothie (1 cup of almond milk, ¼ cup of oats, 1 tablespoon of flaxseed, 1 cup of kale, 1 banana, 1 tablespoon of pure maple syrup).

Snack: Carrot sticks with nut butter.

Lunch: Strawberry, avocado, almond and kale salad. (massage the kale leaves with fresh squeezed lemon until they start to wilt and then assemble your salad).

Snack: Tomatoes, cucumber, mozzarella, and basil drizzled with extra virgin olive oil and balsamic reduction.

Dinner: Burgers with baked sweet potato fries, and mixed greens. Make sure the meat you use for the patty is lean.

Saturday (meatless)

Breakfast: Baked oats with apples and nut butter.

Snack: A mandarin orange and almonds.

Lunch: Black bean and quinoa bowl with spinach, bell peppers, broccoli, tomato, and sliced avocado.

Snack: A small sliver of dark chocolate and 1/2 cup of fresh berries.

Dinner: Whole-wheat pasta with tomatoes, spinach, onions, and mushroom tossed in extra virgin olive oil and nutritional yeast.

Sunday

Breakfast: Avocado toast with sesame seeds and sprouts paired with an apple.

Snack: Strawberry Smoothie (blend together ½ cup of almond milk, ½ cup of strawberries, and 1 tablespoon of nut butter).

Lunch: Cobb salad.

Snack: 12 Almonds

Dinner: Shepherd's Pie (add in extra carrots, peas, onions, and bell peppers).

7-Day Meal Plan (Five Meatless Days)

Monday (meatless)

Breakfast: Strawberry Pineapple Smoothie (blend together ¾ cup of almond milk, ½ cup of strawberries, ½ cup of pineapple, 1 cup of kale or spinach, and 1 tablespoon of almond butter).

Snack: A cup of Greek yogurt with blueberries.

Lunch: Greek salad (cucumber, tomatoes, onions, olives, and feta cheese drizzled with extra virgin olive oil and balsamic vinegar) and an apple.

Snack: Avocado toast.

Dinner: Roasted chickpeas and vegetables with leafy greens and a baked sweet potato.

Tuesday (meatless)

Breakfast: Black bean, bell pepper, and pepper jack cheese burrito with a banana.

Snack: Apple slices and a tablespoon of nut butter.

Lunch: Minestrone soup (made with vegetable broth).

Snack: Raw vegetables with hummus.

Dinner: Tofu pad thai.

Wednesday

Breakfast: Scrambled eggs with mushrooms, spinach, and onions; add a slice of whole-grain toast on the side.

Snack: Half a cup of strawberries and a banana.

Lunch: Lentil soup.

Snack: A pear and a quarter cup of walnuts.

Dinner: Baked salmon, sautéed spinach, and brown rice.

Thursday (meatless)

Breakfast: Oats (made with almond milk) topped with walnuts and fresh fruit.

Snack: Tropical Smoothie (blend together ½ cup of almond milk, ½ cup of strawberries, ½ cup of pineapple, 1 cup of kale or spinach, and ½ tablespoon nut butter).

Lunch: Spicy buffalo cauliflower bowls topped with avocado and a green Tahini dressing.

Snack: Celery sticks with nut butter.

Dinner: Eggplant parmesan served with whole-grain pasta and steamed vegetables.

Friday (meatless)

Breakfast: Green Smoothie (1 cup of almond milk, ¾ cup of oats, 1 tablespoon of flaxseed, 1 cup of kale, 1 banana, 1 tablespoon of pure maple syrup).

Snack: Apple nachos (apple slices topped with melted dark chocolate, nuts, pureed strawberries, and melted nut butter).

Lunch: Strawberry, avocado, almond, and kale salad. (Massage the kale leaves with fresh squeezed lemon until they start to wilt and then assemble your salad).

Snack: Tomatoes, cucumber, mozzarella, and basil drizzled with extra virgin olive oil and balsamic reduction.

Dinner: Black Bean burgers with baked sweet potato fries and mixed greens.

Saturday

Breakfast: Baked oats with apples and nut butter.

Snack: A mandarin orange and almonds.

Lunch: Garden pizza (cauliflower or broccoli crust topped with bell pepper, avocado, tomatoes, mushroom, onions and any other vegetables you enjoy. Drizzle with a fat-free or homemade ranch dressing).

Snack: Fresh dates and nuts

Dinner: Whole-wheat pasta with tomatoes, spinach, onions, and mushrooms tossed in a bolognese sauce.

Sunday (meatless)

Breakfast: Avocado toast with sesame seeds, sprouts, and an apple.

Snack: Strawberry Smoothie (blend together ½ cup of almond milk, ½ cup of strawberries, and 1 tablespoon of nut butter).

Lunch: Falafels with mixed greens and a banana.

Snack: Roasted chickpeas and a half cup of fresh melon.

Dinner: Mushroom Wellinton with cauliflower mash.

Chapter 5:

FODMAP Diet

FODMAP is short for fermentable oligosaccharides, disaccharides, monosaccharides, and polyols. FODMAPs are different types of carbohydrates that can cause bloating, gas, and other digestive issues along with inflammation. A FODMAP diet helps eliminate those foods that trigger digestive problems. This diet is ideal for those who want to take control over their digestive issues while losing weight. Read on to learn more about how to get started, benefits, and more.

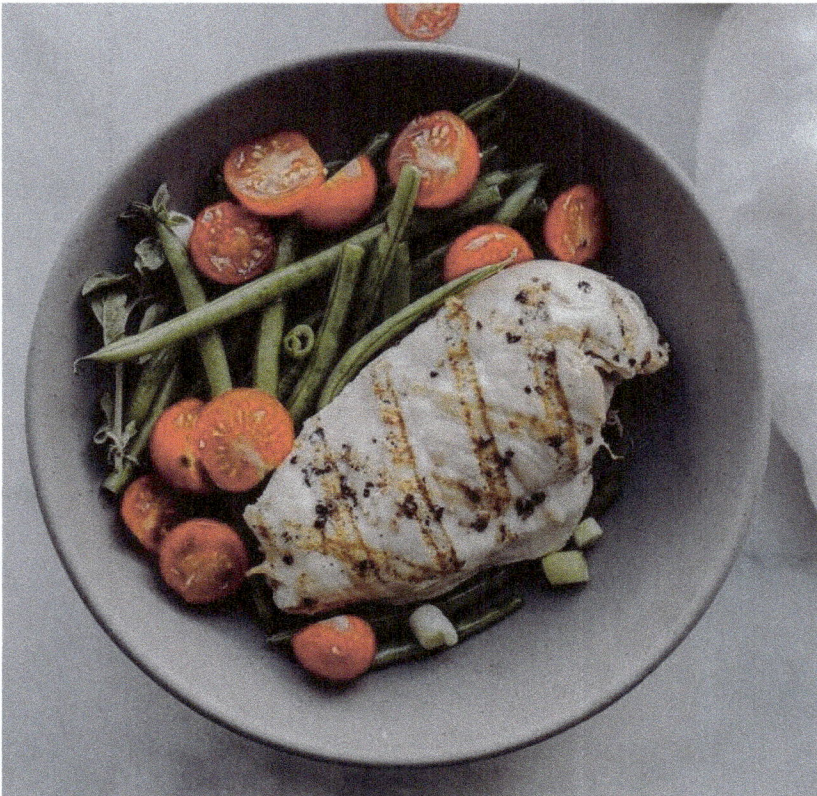

What Is the FODMAP Diet?

The FODMAP diet is categorized as a low-carb diet, but it serves a much bigger purpose than limiting carb intake. The FODMAP or low-FODMAP diet is ideal for those who have serious food sensitivities or digestive issues like irritable bowel syndrome (IBS). This diet is a three-stage plan that eliminates the most common food irritants or high FODMAP foods. Over the three stages, you will slowly add higher FODMAP foods back into your diet to pinpoint which ones trigger symptoms and how much you can tolerate. The stages are broken down as follows:

Stage One: The Elimination Stage

In the first stage, you will eliminate all high FODMAP carbs:

- Fructose: including fruits, honey, agave, and high fructose corn syrup. Dried fruits and concentrated fruit juices are also in this category.
- Lactose: including dairy (from cows, goats, and sheep), yogurt, ice cream, and soft cheese (cottage cheese, cream cheese, ricotta, and mascarpone).
- Fructans: including many grains like rye and wheat. Many vegetables contain fructans like; onions, garlic, cabbage, asparagus, brussel sprouts, eggplant, okra, leeks, shallots, fennel, and broccoli.
- Galatians: including legumes, beans, lentils, soybeans, and chickpeas.
- Polyols: including sugar alcohols and pitted fruits or fruits with seeds like apricots, avocados, cherries, peaches, plums, figs, and pears. Vegetables like green bell peppers, mushrooms, and sweet corn contain polyols. You also want to eliminate sweeteners like sorbitol and xylitol.

Stick with this elimination for a minimum of two weeks and no more than six. During these weeks, you will be consuming only foods considered low FODMAPs, which include:

- lettuce
- carrots
- cucumbers
- celery
- green beans
- bok choy
- zucchini
- kiwi
- mandarins
- oranges
- pineapple
- cantaloupe
- strawberries
- gouda
- parmesan
- feta
- almond milk
- lactose-free milk
- soy milk (made from soy protein)
- firm tofu
- tempeh
- eggs
- cooked meats
- poultry
- seafood
- oats
- quinoa or pasta
- wheat/rye/barley free breads
- spelt bread
- dark chocolate
- maple syrup

- macadamia nuts
- pumpkin seeds
- walnuts

After sticking with low FODMAP foods, any symptoms of your digestive issues should subside or be completely gone. Many find their symptoms improve immediately, and others do not notice a change until after six weeks. If symptoms are still persistent and unchanged after six weeks there may be other medical issues that need to be addressed. Consult with your primary care physician to address your concerns and other treatment options available. If you have no irritation or digestive problems for a week, you can move on to stage two.

Stage Two: The Reintroduction Stage

This stage takes the longest amount of time. Most people will continue to reintroduce foods for twelve weeks. During this stage, you go through a list of the high FODMAP food groups; add one group and one food from that group at a time. For example, you may begin with the lactose FODMAPs and start by adding in cow's milk. You would start with a small amount of cow's milk just once a day. Next, you will increase the serving size slightly and repeat this the following day. Each food will be introduced over a three-day period which will allow you to monitor symptoms or unpleasant reactions.

It is recommended that when you first begin the introduction stage, you stick with only adding foods that are high in just one FODMAP category—like milk—as opposed to starting with a food that is high in two or more FODMAPS like apples and wheat.

Stage Three: The Personalization Stage

In the third stage, you will create meals based on the information gained during the second stage. You'll know which foods you want to avoid completely and which you can tolerate a moderate amount. The process can be cumbersome but is well worth the time once you know which foods you should avoid.

Benefits

Learning which foods can cause digestive issues can help you understand why you may have struggled with your weight up until now. Digestive issues can lead to weight gain and can keep you from being active. While a Low-FODMAP diet is not easy to sustain long-term, it does help you identify foods you should permanently eliminate or cut back on in your diet. There are additional benefits that you should know about that may entice you to start a FODMAP diet.

Helps Relieve Symptoms of Irritable Bowel Syndrome (IBS) and Inflammatory Bowel Syndrome

The low-FODMAP diet was created to help treat IBS and digestive distress. Various research has proven that short-chain carbohydrates—those that are eliminated during phase one of high-FODMAPs—can not be properly absorbed by most people. This poor absorption triggers IBS symptoms along with other digestive complications. Removing these foods helps alleviate IBS symptoms.

Helps Identify Foods That Cause Digestive Issues

Through the reintroduction phase, high FODMAP foods are slowly added back into the diet, both in volume and frequency. Slowly reintroducing foods in this manner helps individuals determine what foods trigger symptoms and how much of certain foods they can tolerate without exhibiting symptoms. Though this process is lengthy, it allows individuals to create a diet that best works with their bodies. It also allows individuals to understand that not every food needs to be completely cut out; they may be able to tolerate a small or moderate amount without symptoms.

Can Help Manage Crohn's Disease

Crohn's disease and IBS have similar symptoms which make the low-FODMAP diet an effective way to help manage the symptoms that accompany Crohn's disease. The low-FODMAP diet can help alleviate cramping, gas, bloating, and irregular bowel movements like diarrhea (Halas-Liang, 2016).

Cons

The low-FODMAP diet is essentially only recommended for those who suffer from digestive issues. This is not a traditional weight loss diet plan, though individuals who go through each stage will see weight loss as many carbs and sweeteners are being eliminated for weeks at a time.

This is not a long-term diet plan. The goal by the end of the third stage is that you will be back to eating many of the foods you ate previously with the exception of those that cause severe digestive distress.

This diet is very restrictive during the first stage. Like other diets followed in phases, it is hard to stick with. Not following the plan precisely in the beginning will not provide the benefits it promises. The second stage also has its challenges. Having to slowly reintroduce foods one at a time requires a great deal of patience to complete properly. Trying to speed up this process by adding foods too quickly can trigger digestive issues to reappear without fully understanding what is causing them.

This diet is not easy to modify. Those who are vegan, vegetarian, or have other food restrictions may find it hard to adhere to the guidelines in each stage.

Pregnant women and young children should not partake in the low FODMAP diet because of the many dietary restrictions. Until you reach phase three of the plan you are limiting your calorie intake a great deal because most low-FODMAP foods naturally have fewer calories. While this is great for weight loss, it is not recommended while pregnant when your body needs more calories to support your growing baby. Young children also need to consume more calories for proper growth which they may not get enough of in phases one or two. Aside from the calorie intake, eliminating things like dairy, fruits, and grains cut out important nutrients your body needs.

Getting Started

Getting help as you go through each stage will make sticking to the FODMAP diet much easier. Luckily, there is plenty of helpful information available for the whole diet plan. A valuable app to use is the Monash FODMAP App. It provides you with a list of foods to eliminate during the first stage and recommends the right foods to add during the second stage. It is also designed with a food diary feature that lets you record any symptoms or irritation that those foods may cause.

7-Day Meal Plan

Monday

Breakfast: Oatmeal made with almond milk and topped with blueberries.

Lunch: Grilled chicken salad with balsamic vinegar topped with feta and fresh strawberries.

Snack: Fruit Smoothie (blend together ½ a banana, 1 cup of almond milk, and 1 tablespoon of almond butter, add ice for a thicker smoothie).

Dinner: Gluten-free Margherita pizza.

Snack: Fresh pineapple chunks.

Tuesday

Breakfast: Spinach, tomato, and feta omelet.

Lunch: Quinoa salad with baked chicken and zucchini.

Snack: Walnuts.

Dinner: Chili (made with lentils instead of beans).

Snack: Orange slices and a small square of dark chocolate (80% cacao).

Wednesday

Breakfast: Overnight oats with almond butter and bananas.

Lunch: Tuna salad over salad greens.

Snack: Chia Smoothie (blend together 1 cup almond milk, ½ cup frozen blueberries, 1 tablespoon chia seeds, 1 tablespoon maple syrup and ice for desired thickness).

Dinner: Pork fried rice (made with brown rice).

Snack: Lactose-free frozen yogurt.

Thursday

Breakfast: Cheddar cheese and red bell pepper scramble.

Lunch: Vegetable soup (be sure there are no beans).

Snack: Roasted chickpeas.

Dinner: Baked salmon served with roasted potatoes and carrots.

Snack: Raspberry sorbet.

Friday

Breakfast: Flaxseed Smoothie (blend together 1 ½ cups of almond milk, 1 cup of frozen strawberries, 1 tablespoon flaxseed meal, 1 tablespoon almond butter, and ice for a thicker smoothie).

Lunch: Egg salad served with greens.

Snack: Plain popcorn.

Dinner: Beef stew.

Snack: Fresh fruit (strawberries, pineapples, blueberries).

Saturday

Breakfast: 2 hard-boiled eggs and ½ cup of cantaloupe.

Lunch: Grilled chicken salad.

Snack: Macadamia nuts and lactose-free yogurt.

Dinner: Eggplant parmesan (made with gluten-free breadcrumbs) served with zucchini noodles or baked potatoes.

Snack: Banana slices and peanut butter.

Sunday

Breakfast: Blueberry oat muffins.

Lunch: Vegetable stir fry with brown rice noodles.

Snack: Spelt toast with nut butter.

Dinner: Baked chicken, quinoa, and sweet potato bowls.

Snack: Strawberry sorbet.

Chapter 6:

Gluten-Free Diet

Gluten free has been a craze in the dieting world. You will find plenty of products on the market claiming to be gluten-free. Many people buy them in hopes of managing their weight and improving their health. Unfortunately, gluten has obtained a bad reputation because of misleading and biased claims that say gluten is bad for you. A gluten-free diet does have its benefits but it is not beneficial for everyone. You can lose weight by cutting out products that contain gluten, but you need to ensure you are getting the right balance of nutrients and vitamins to maintain optimal health. In this chapter, you will learn what gluten-free means, why you might consider a gluten-free diet, and other benefits of decreasing your gluten intake.

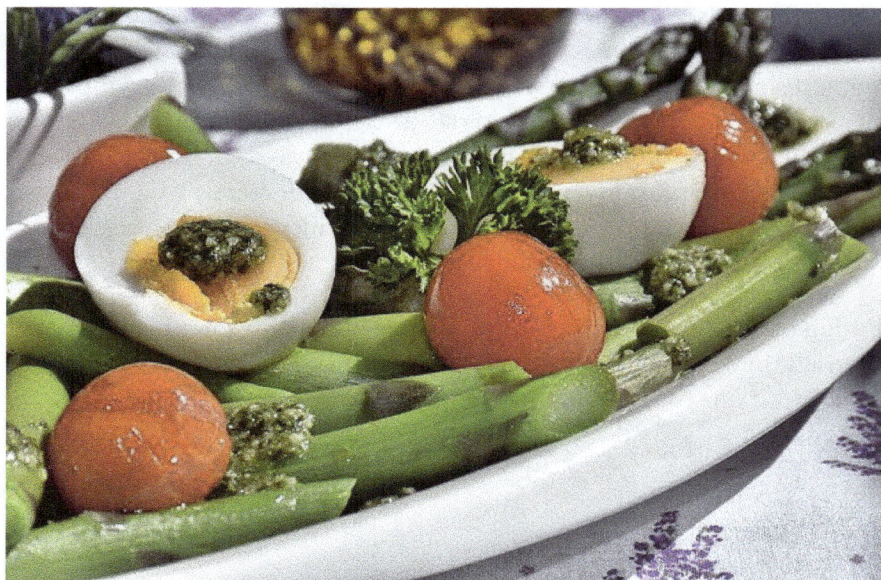

What Is the Gluten-Free Diet?

Gluten is a protein found in grains and is added to many foods to give them more texture. It is also used as a thickener and binding agent and can even be used to add color to some items. Many people think gluten-free means only eliminating carbs like pasta, cereal, and pizza dough, but other products can contain gluten as well. Soy sauce, ice cream, medications, and some alcohol like beer are just a few unexpected items containing gluten.

Those with celiac disease must eat a gluten-free diet because of the negative way their body responds to gluten. Celiac disease is a type of autoimmune disorder where the body attacks its own cells. When individuals with celiac disease consume gluten, the body attacks the small intestines. If the damage continues to occur in the small intestines they are unable to absorb nutrients properly. Celiac disease is hereditary, so if someone in your family has it you have a greater chance of developing it. The condition can occur at any age and if untreated can lead to serious health conditions.

Individuals who are sensitive to gluten will often see an improvement with their symptoms. Gluten sensitivity or intolerance is not as serious as Celiac disease but causes a wide range of ailments. Those with this condition will feel bloated, gassy, tired, nauseous, and even become sick after consuming gluten. If you suffer from any of these symptoms, a gluten-free diet can help you avoid discomforts after eating. Keep in mind; however, you may just have an intolerance to certain foods that contain gluten and may be fine consuming other forms of gluten. It is also a good idea to talk to your doctor about your concerns before eliminating all gluten from your diet.

Understand what grains have gluten in them and which do not naturally have gluten. Gluten-containing grains include wheat, barley, and rye. Grains that are naturally gluten-free include:

- buckwheat
- corn
- millet
- wild rice
- soy
- arrowroot

- flax
- teff

Oats are also gluten-free but have a greater risk of cross-contamination. If another grain is manufactured in the same facility as the oats, there is a chance that some of those grains or particles of the grains can get mixed up with the oats. These particles can be transferred from employees, through the air, or left on the machines if the same equipment is used to process the grains.

Always double-check the labels. Just because a product is labeled gluten-free does not mean you should eat it. Many gluten-free products contain high amounts of sodium, fat, and sugar, which are associated with a greater risk of heart disease.

You also need to check the label for gluten variations. On food labels, wheat gluten can be listed as:

- durum
- kamut
- spelt
- einkorn
- enriched flours
- farina
- graham flour
- self-rising flour
- phosphate flour
- semolina

If you are looking at gluten-free products do not just take the label as a safe bet. Always check the ingredients. Many products can get away with being labeled gluten-free but may have gluten additives.

Foods you should stock up on when going gluten-free include:

- fresh meat, poultry, seafood, fish, and eggs
- fresh fruits and vegetables
- frozen fruits and vegetables

- corn flour, cornmeal, polenta, and grits
- basmati or brown rice
- arrowroot
- buckwheat, flaxseed, millet, quinoa
- coconut flour
- almond flour
- vinegar
- oil
- spices
- herbs

If you do have a gluten intolerance or celiac disease, it is important to avoid cross-contamination in your own home. If you are the only person going gluten-free you will need to come up with a system to keep the gluten and gluten-free items separated. Also consider your kitchen appliances, tools, and utensils. The toaster can easily contaminate gluten-free foods with gluten if both items are used in the same toaster. It may sound extreme but even the smallest amount of gluten can trigger flare-ups.

Benefits

If you have an issue with gluten, eliminating it from your diet can help you enjoy your food more. There are a few other reasons you may want to consider limiting your gluten consumption.

Lose Weight

A gluten-free diet can help you lose and manage weight. A gluten-free diet eliminates many processed foods known to cause weight gain. Many processed foods lack nutrients but are high in calories. When you eliminate these from your diet, you will see some weight loss and may even feel better because you will be replacing these foods with nutrient-rich foods like vegetables.

Regulate Digestion

Gluten is a common trigger for digestive issues like bloating, gas, constipation, and cramps. By removing gluten from your diet you may find your stomach issues decrease and even disappear.

Reduce Inflammation

Chronic inflammation is directly influenced by what we eat. If you suffer from conditions like rheumatoid arthritis or notice pain, swelling, redness, or heat radiating from your joints this can be a sign of inflammation. When the digestive tract can not properly process food—which is common with gluten—this can trigger an inflammatory response in the body. While an inflammatory response is essential when there is a threat, injury, or infection in the body, an inflammatory response to food can cause long-term complications. Those who have chronic inflammation and eliminate gluten from their diet often find relief from these pains and can manage their condition in a natural way.

Cons

If you do not have a gluten intolerance, going gluten-free can result in losing out on nutrients your body needs. Whole grains that contain gluten also contain a significant source of fiber and other macronutrients. Whole grains are also essential for a healthy heart and help regulate blood sugar levels. Removing processed foods from your diet can give you the same health benefits of a gluten-free diet without losing out on valuable nutrients.

When you switch to a gluten-free diet you may experience dizziness, nausea, anxiety, and even depression. Individuals who drastically switch from eating an excessive amount of gluten to no gluten at all are likely to have these symptoms for a few weeks until the body adjusts.

Cutting out all gluten-containing foods can also lead to developing digestive issues. Many foods containing gluten also provide a significant source of fiber. Not getting enough fiber can lead to poor gut health and result in irregular bowel movements, irregular blood sugar levels, and constipation. Fiber also helps suppress appetite. Most people who consume a Western diet do not get sufficient fiber which could be the cause for any digestive issues they may be experiencing.

Fiber also helps with appetite control. Skipping out on eating high-fiber foods can cause you to feel more hungry throughout the day and lead to overeating. Those considering a gluten-free diet need to carefully choose gluten-free foods that contain enough fiber to help them feel satiated throughout the day to reduce the risk of weight gain.

Getting Started

The most important thing to remember when going gluten-free is that it is a learning process. It is important to teach yourself how to read labels on food packages, how to order in a restaurant, how to cook healthy and delicious meals from home, and how to embrace gluten-free as a lifestyle.

Unless you have a medical diagnosis that requires you to go gluten-free, having a little gluten in your diet is not going to break the scale. Find options that don't contain gluten to replace those that do or, learn what products are naturally gluten free. You want to avoid whole wheat or whole grain bread but you can still consume easy to find grains like quinoa, wild rice, and millet.

Invest in a quality blender and food processor. Since many sauces, jams, and condiments available in the store have hidden gluten, you should consider learning how to make these yourself. Fresh fruits and vegetables are gluten free and serve as the foundation for many of these items you will not be able to buy.

Avoid buying flavored dairy. Regular dairy like plain yogurt, milk, and cottage cheese should not contain gluten. Flavored products like chocolate milk, strawberry yogurt, or cottage cheese with fruit may contain gluten.

7-Day Meal Plan

Monday

Breakfast: Breakfast Quinoa (with blueberries, raspberries, and toasted coconut).

Lunch: Zucchini noodles with bolognese sauce.

Dinner: Polenta with roasted vegetables and two fried eggs.

Snack: Raw veggies (carrots, celery, bell peppers, cucumbers).

Tuesday

Breakfast: Banana pancakes (mix together a banana and two eggs, then cook in a frying pan).

Lunch: Tuna and chickpeas over leafy greens with a balsamic vinaigrette.

Dinner: Baked chicken with steamed cauliflower and broccoli with sweet potato fries.

Snack: An apple and a cup of raspberries.

Wednesday

Breakfast: Nonfat plain Greek yogurt with blueberries and walnuts.

Lunch: Tomato soup with grilled cheese using cloud bread (made from egg whites).

Dinner: Grilled salmon with steamed green beans and roasted potatoes.

Snack: A cup of raspberries and two tablespoons of unsalted peanuts.

Thursday

Breakfast: Omelet made with bacon, broccoli, onions, and cheddar cheese.

Lunch: Turkey, cheese, tomatoes, and cucumber wrapped in a large lettuce leaf with a side of fresh fruit.

Dinner: Grilled chicken breast, steamed broccoli, carrots, and a small side of quinoa.

Snack: Tropical Smoothie (1 cup of spinach, ½ cup of water, 1 banana, 1 teaspoon of shredded coconut, ½ cup of mango, and ½ cup of pineapple).

Friday

Breakfast: Gluten-free steel cut oats with banana and nut butter.

Lunch: Steamed asparagus with tuna and roasted red potatoes.

Dinner: Ultimate stuffed baked potatoes (stuff with chicken, onions, peppers, cheddar cheese, or any other vegetables you prefer).

Snack: Low-fat plain Greek yogurt and apples drizzled with maple syrup.

Saturday

Breakfast: Two eggs with bacon and a side of fresh fruit.

Lunch: Avocado salad (avocado, cherry tomatoes, cucumber, and red onions) topped with shrimp and served in a lettuce bowl. Drizzle with a lemon and red wine vinaigrette.

Dinner: Spaghetti squash with bolognese sauce and sautéed spinach.

Snack: Grapes, pecans, and celery.

Sunday

Breakfast: Peanut Butter Banana Smoothie (blend together 1 cup of spinach, ½ cup of almond milk, 1 banana, 1 tablespoon of nut butter, and 1 teaspoon of maple syrup).

Lunch: Cauliflower rice bowl with grilled chicken, spinach, tomatoes, and avocado.

Dinner: Pork tenderloin and mixed green salad with a citrus vinaigrette.

Snack: A hard-boiled egg, string cheese, and pears.

Chapter 7:

Intermittent Fasting Diet

Intermittent fasting is less of a diet and more of a new way of eating. While there are suggestions as to what to eat there is more emphasis on when to eat. You will learn that an intermittent fasting diet can be an addition to any healthy eating plan and many find great success with losing weight and managing weight with this approach. There are many ways you can incorporate intermittent fasting into your new diet plan. You may be surprised to learn that you already adhere to an intermittent fasting lifestyle.

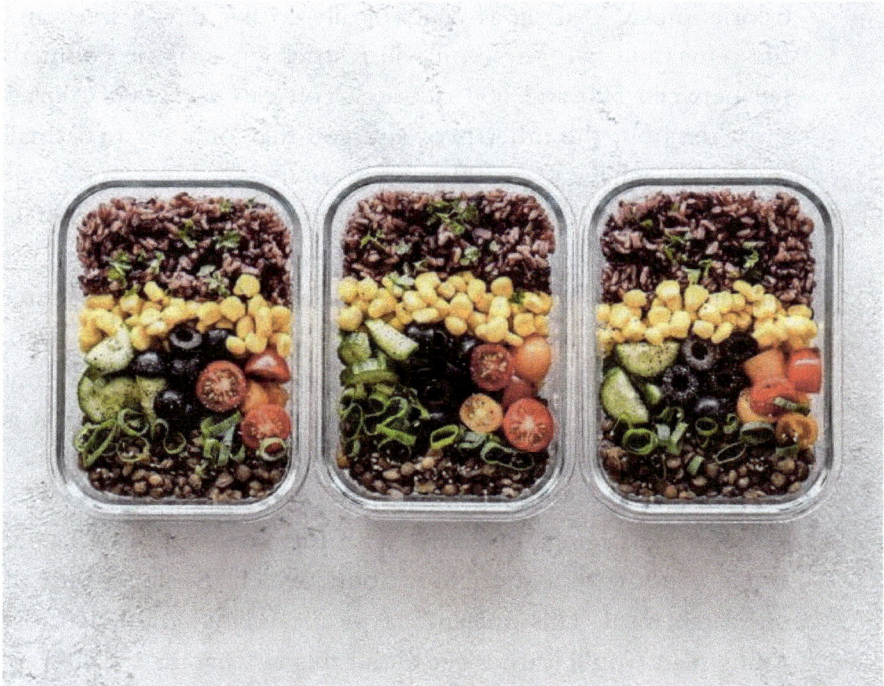

What Is the Intermittent Fasting Diet?

Intermittent fasting has become a popular eating plan. There are a few ways you can adopt an intermittent fasting diet. One is to restrict the timeframe you eat during your day and another is to restrict your calorie intake on specific days. With these two approaches, intermittent fasting can be completely customizable, making it easier to find a diet plan that fits best with your lifestyle. Some intermittent fasting approaches to consider include:

- 16/8 fasting plan- With this approach you limit your eating window to only eight hours a day and fast for the remaining 16. For example, your first meal can be at 10 a.m., and your last meal would be at 6 pm.

- 5:2 fasting plan- With this approach you are restricting your calorie intake. You eat as you typically do five days a week and the remaining two days you will restrict your calorie count to fall between 500 and 600 calories. You can eat 2,000 calories most days but the other two days you may only eat two small meals that equal 250 to 300 calories each.

- 24 hour fast- With a 24-hour intermittent fasting diet you fast for a full 24 hours once or twice a week. For example, if you eat dinner around 6:30 p.m., on Friday your next meal will be after 6:30 p.m., on Saturday. During the 24-hour fast, you can drink water, black coffee, or other zero-calorie drinks but you cannot eat any solid foods. If you are going too fast for two days it is important not to plan them back to back, meaning you do not want to fast for 48-hours straight.

- The warrior fasting approach- With this fast, you restrict your eating window to a short four hours, which usually consist of one large meal. This one meal typically follows the Paleo diet eating plan (you'll learn more about this in Chapter 13). During the rest of the day; however, you are allowed to eat a small number of raw fruits and vegetables.

Benefits

Aside from weight-loss, there are many other reasons people stick with a fasting plan. Intermittent fasting has shown promising results in studies that pertain to various aspects of one's health and overall well-being. Below you will learn a few of the key ways intermittent fasting can help you lose weight and feel more energized.

Reduce the Risk of Insulin Resistance and Type 2 Diabetes

Though more studies need to be conducted, there is the promise that intermittent fasting can improve insulin sensitivity in those who are obese or at greater risk of developing type 2 diabetes. A preliminary review of studies comparing intermittent fasting to calorie restriction diets has shown to reduce fasting insulin levels and fasting glucose levels (Barnosky et al., 2014). When insulin and glucose levels are low it means your body is not creating insulin or using glucose. High insulin levels are an indicator of prediabetes but can also cause a wide range of other issues. Lower HDL cholesterol levels, high LDL cholesterol levels, storing excess fat, and increased inflammation can all occur when insulin levels are too high. These conditions also put one at greater risk of heart disease and cardiovascular disease. Intermittent fasting can help bring down insulin levels and lower the risk of type 2 diabetes and other health problems.

Simplifies Healthy Eating

You do not need to count calories or follow a specific list of things you can and can not eat. Since intermittent fasting is about when you eat, it can make eating healthier easier for most. Those who want more flexibility with their healthy eating plan may enjoy the freedom intermittent fasting provides. However, one needs to ensure their eating window is focused on consuming fresh fruits and vegetables and more whole foods instead of easy-to-grab processed foods.

Other Advantages

There are additional studies that have been conducted that show how intermittent fasting may benefit some, but not all individuals. Additional benefits you may experience from intermittent fasting include:

- Improved skin and hair.
- Improved brain health.
- Protection against certain cancers.
- Increased life-expectancy.
- Reduced LDL (bad) cholesterol levels.
- Lowered triglyceride levels.
- Reduced inflammation.
- Lowered risk of heart disease.
- Protection against Alzheimer's disease.

These additional benefits are promising, but keep in mind the research done on these benefits focuses on short-term fasting and some studies are inconclusive.

Cons

Intermittent Fasting is a tool that can help you consume fewer calories. However, if you eat high-calorie foods and unhealthy foods during your eating windows you will not reap the benefits from fasting.

Women may not benefit from intermittent fasting as much as men. When women fast, their bodies are hardwired to conserve energy and store fat as it anticipates when your next meal will be. This causes stress to the body which releases cortisol (the stress hormone). When the body produces more cortisol it triggers the production of ghrelin, the hunger hormone. Binge eating is common for women because of this extra production of ghrelin.

Fasting can also have a negative impact on the reproductive system and fertility. Women should be aware that fasting can cause changes in their menstrual cycle; in a few women, their periods have stopped all together. Women who are trying to conceive, are pregnant, or are breastfeeding should avoid intermittent fasting.

Extreme hunger is another common side effect when fasting. While these hunger pangs tend to subside as your body adjusts, there are a few people where extreme hunger persists.

When you are starting out on Intermittent Fasting, it is common to have some brain fog or decrease brain performance. You may also feel more weak or fatigued than you used to. For many, these side effects are temporary.

Those with diabetes, irregular blood sugar, low blood pressure, are on medications, have a history of eating disorders, or those who are underweight should speak to their primary care physician first.

Getting Started

Start out with a 14 or 16 hours fast. Many people already fast for this amount of time as much of their fasting time takes place while they sleep. Alternatively, you may also begin by skipping a meal here and there. You do not need to follow a structured fasting plan, you just need to find an approach that works for your lifestyle.

Before you choose a fasting plan, know what your goals are. Many people begin fasting to lose weight while others just want to improve their health. Having a clear goal in mind will help you identify which approach will allow you to reach your goals.

Stick with one fasting approach for at least a month before trying another or deciding it isn't for you. You might struggle at first with going an extended period of time without eating but if you only try it once, you cannot know for sure if it will benefit you. It is best to commit to one approach before jumping ship and trying another.

Keep yourself hydrated. Drinking water can help combat hunger, making it easier to commit to your fasting plan. It is also common for people who are fasting to forget to drink plenty of water when they are not eating which can lead to dehydration.

Stock up on healthy foods. After fasting for any period of time it is more common for individuals to binge on whatever foods are most convenient. Binging on unhealthy foods is not going to help you reach your weight loss or healthy lifestyle goals. While fasting can make eating healthy easier because it minimizes the meals you have to plan, you should still plan out your meals to avoid overeating on junk and unfulfilling foods.

Choose foods that are high in fiber and eat plenty of vegetables during your feasting window. These foods will not only supply you with plenty of nutrients, but they will also help you feel fuller for longer.

7-Day Meal Plan (16/8 Intermittent Fasting Plan)

For this plan you want to ensure you keep your first and last meal within an eight hour window. An example of this would be:

- 10 a.m.,- breakfast
- 12 p.m.,- snack
- 2 p.m.,- lunch
- 4 p.m.,- snack
- 6 p.m.,- dinner

If you rise early and know you need food in your system to function right away, your day might look like this:

- 7 a.m.,- breakfast
- 9 a.m.,- snack
- 11 a.m.,- lunch
- 1 p.m.,- snack
- 3 p.m.,- dinner

You can use the above outlines as a guide to creating your own fasting and eating windows with the following meal plan. Sticking with a consistent time frame will make transitioning to an intermittent fasting plan easier. Try to avoid inconsistency; if your first meal begins at 10 a.m., some days and 6 a.m., other days you will not see desired results. If you need to switch up your time frame, it is important that you stick with the same fasting hours—in this case 16 hours. Breaking your fast early will minimize the benefits.

Monday

Breakfast: Oatmeal with banana and cinnamon.

Snack: Hard boiled egg and avocado slices on whole-wheat toast.

Lunch: Roasted chicken with strawberry and spinach salad.

Snack: Cottage cheese with fresh berries or peaches.

Dinner: Pork chops with roasted potatoes and steamed vegetables.

Tuesday

Breakfast: Spinach and mushroom omelet with toast and an orange.

Snack: Banana Smoothie (blend together 1 cup of milk, ½ cup of yogurt, 1 banana, ½ cup spinach, 1 tablespoon flaxseed, and ½ cup of mixed berries).

Lunch: Brown rice bowl with ground turkey, black beans, salsa, and guacamole.

Snack: Carrots and bell pepper sticks with hummus.

Dinner: Lean steak and vegetable stir-fry.

Wednesday

Breakfast: Scrambled egg on a bagel with tomatoes, lettuce, and avocado.

Snack: Greek yogurt with walnuts and apple slices.

Lunch: Tuna salad on whole-wheat toast and a side of mixed greens.

Snack: Poached pears and pecans.

Dinner: Chili with cornbread.

Thursday

Breakfast: Quinoa breakfast bowl with apples and cinnamon.

Snack: Fruit and cheese.

Lunch: Burger (with or without bread or cheese; feel free to add your favorite toppings) with fries and a piece of fruit.

Snack: Salsa and chips.

Dinner: Zucchini noodles with turkey meatballs.

Friday

Breakfast: Vegetable frittata and a side of sliced melon.

Snack: Yogurt with fresh fruit and granola.

Lunch: Grilled chicken with lettuce, bell pepper, cucumber, and celery in a whole-wheat pita with a half cup of fresh strawberries.

Snack: Banana and apple slices with a tablespoon of almond butter on whole-wheat toast.

Dinner: Herb crusted salmon with roasted cauliflower, asparagus, and sweet potato.

Saturday

Breakfast: Fruit, nuts, and yogurt parfait.

Snack: Tomato, cucumber, and mozzarella.

Lunch: Shrimp fried rice.

Snack: Nut butter, banana, and chia seed pudding.

Dinner: Grilled steak salad with a side of fresh cantaloupe.

Sunday

Breakfast: Breakfast burrito and a half cup of mixed fruit.

Snack: Berry Smoothie (blend together a cup of almond milk, a cup of mixed berries, and a cup of spinach).

Lunch: Chicken zucchini noodle pad thai.

Snack: Hard boiled eggs and a piece of fruit.

Dinner: Beef stew.

7-Day Meal Plan (2 24-Hour Intermittent Fasting Days)

Keep in mind that the first meal after your 24-hour fast should be a fiber rich meal with a lean source of protein. The protein and fiber combination will allow you to fill up on the rich nutrients without the risk of overeating.

Monday

Breakfast: Sausage, egg, and cheese sandwich with an apple.

Snack: Smoothie (blend together 1 cup of milk, ½ cup yogurt, 1 cup of spinach, ½ cup pineapple, ½ cup strawberries, and 1 tablespoon honey).

Lunch: Grilled chicken wrap and sweet potato fries.

Snack: Yogurt with fresh fruit.

Dinner (around 6 p.m.): Pork chops with roasted potatoes and steamed vegetables.

Tuesday

Breakfast: Fast

Snack: Fast

Lunch: Fast

Snack: Fast

Dinner (around 6 p.m.): Lean steak and vegetable stir-fry.

Wednesday

Breakfast: Baked oatmeal with apples, walnuts, and cinnamon.

Snack: Greek yogurt with walnuts and apple slices.

Lunch: Tuna salad on whole-wheat toast and a side of mixed greens.

Snack: Poached pears and pecans.

Dinner: Chili with cornbread.

Thursday

Breakfast: Cinnamon raisin muffins with almond butter and a banana.

Snack: Fruit and cheese.

Lunch: Burrito bowl.

Snack: Turkey and cheese roll ups.

Dinner: Zucchini noodles with turkey meatballs.

Friday

Breakfast: Blueberry pancakes.

Snack: Yogurt with fresh fruit and granola.

Lunch: Grilled chicken with lettuce, bell pepper, cucumber, and celery in a whole-wheat pita with a half cup of fresh strawberries.

Snack: Banana and apple slices with a tablespoon of almond butter on whole-wheat toast.

Dinner (around 6 p.m.): Herb crusted salmon with roasted cauliflower, asparagus, and sweet potatoes.

Saturday

Breakfast: Fast

Snack: Fast

Lunch: Fast

Snack: Fast

Dinner (around 6 p.m.): Grilled steak salad with a side of fresh cantaloupe.

Sunday

Breakfast: Two poached eggs with baked hash browns and turkey bacon.

Snack: Banana Smoothie (blend together 1 cup of milk, ½ cup of yogurt, 1 banana, ½ cup spinach, 1 tablespoon flax seed, and ½ cup of mixed berries).

Lunch: Turkey, spinach, tomatoes, and avocado wrap with a piece of fruit on the side.

Snack: Chocolate chia seed pudding

Dinner: Barbeque ribs with a loaded sweet potato and grilled vegetables.

Chapter 8:

Ketogenic Diet (Keto)

The Ketogenic diet was originally designed to help children who suffered from epileptic seizures. Keto has become highly popularized and is so mainstream now that many companies have created products claiming to be Keto friendly. There is a lot to understand about this diet plan before jumping on the Keto bandwagon.

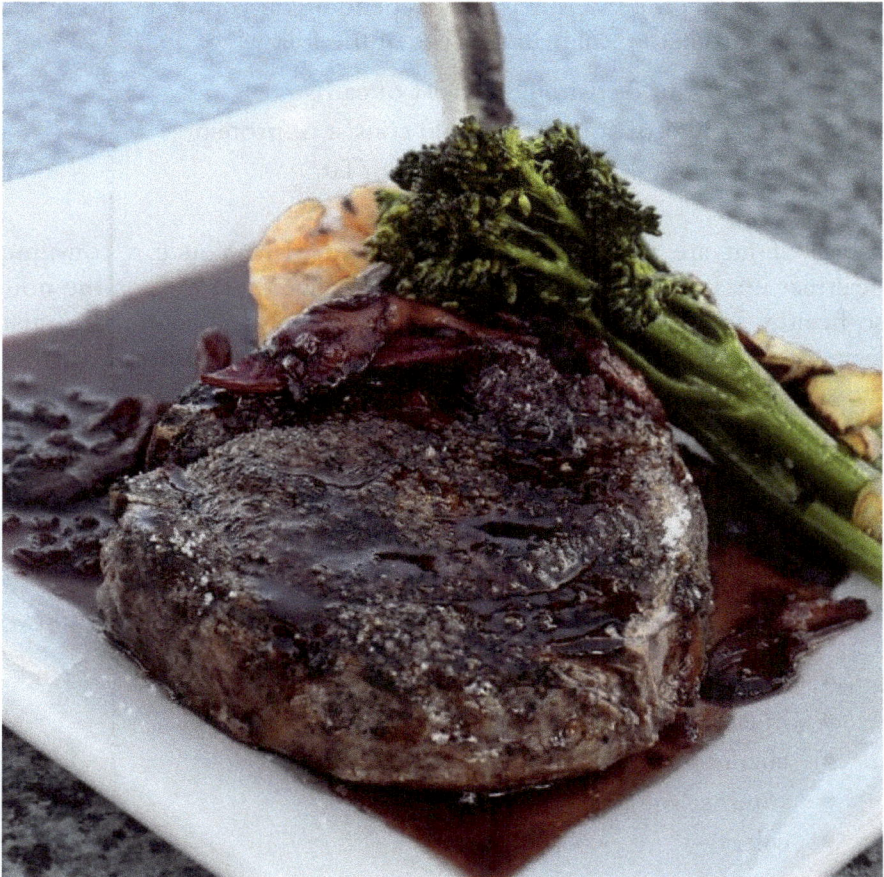

What Is the Ketogenic Diet?

The Keto diet focuses on consuming more protein; as with other low-carb diets, it focuses on consuming more fat as well. The idea behind limiting carbs while increasing fat intake is to put the body in a natural state of ketosis. When the body is in ketosis, the liver begins to produce ketones from stored fat. This process encourages the body to use its stored fat as fuel instead of relying on a steady stream of carbs. Getting the body into ketosis and remaining there is a challenge, though.

On the Keto diet, you are restricting your carb intake to 50 grams or less a day. While the ratios may vary depending on your goals, with this diet a standard keto meal plan consists of the following:

- 5% of your diet should consist of carbs
- 10 to 30% of your diet should consist of protein.
- 75% of your diet should consist of fat.

Types of fat are not restricted on the keto plan. You can consume healthier unsaturated fats like avocado and olive oil as well as the not-so-healthy saturated fats like butter. Protein is also not limited to just lean meats. Bacon, pork, and beef are regularly consumed in higher quantities on the Keto diet. Since many vegetables contain carbs, these are restricted to only a handful including:

- leafy greens (kale, spinach, Swiss chard)
- broccoli
- brussel sprouts
- bell peppers
- garlic
- onions
- mushroom
- cucumbers
- summer squash
- celery

Fruits are eliminated with the exception of berries and these should only be consumed in small portions. There are alternative keto diet plans to consider as well.

The cyclical ketogenic diet includes carb refeed days. This is ideal for athletes looking to build muscle mass. Keep in mind, refeed days are limited to two a week and these will take the body out of ketosis.

The targeted ketogenic diet is also primarily used by extreme athletes. With this diet, you are allowed to add carbs around your workout times. The carbs consumed are burned during your workout so it is less likely that the body will come out of ketosis.

The targeted ketogenic diet is similar to the standard keto plan with the exception that it increases total protein to 35% and lowers fat intake to 60%.

There are many people who partake in both the keto diet and intermittent fasting diet. The idea behind this is that fasting will help speed up the process and put the body in ketosis faster.

Benefits

As with any low-carb diet, you are bound to experience a wide range of benefits. The Keto diet provides the same benefits that any other low-carb diet provides but may also help you lose stubborn weight and improve other aspects of your health.

Helps You Lose Weight

The keto diet cuts out high-calorie carbs that lead to weight gain. Many studies show that a keto diet is effective for rapid weight loss, though keeping the weight off long-term is still questionable on a keto diet. The keto diet also helps reprogram your body to burn the stored fat it has instead of relying on instant fuel from simple carbs that many of us consume.

Lowers Blood Sugar Levels

A keto diet can help those with type 2 diabetes drastically lower blood sugar levels in the short term. Keep in mind, cholesterol levels are shown to increase in individuals on a keto diet which can put those with diabetes at even greater risk of heart complications. The increase in cholesterol has been shown to drop after a few months on the diet.

May Improve Brain Health

Studies have been conducted to identify whether the Keto diet can have a positive impact on other brain-related issues. The brain does perform more efficiently when it is getting its energy from glucose; but as one ages, the brain loses its ability to properly transform glucose into energy. Instead, it can utilize ketones for energy. Older individuals can help keep the brain sharp on a keto diet as the body produces enough ketones to keep the brain fueled.

Studies have also shown that a keto diet can help protect brain cells and reduce the risk of brain degeneration that can lead to Parkinson's or Alzheimer's (Winters, 2020). Another brain benefit the keto diet has been shown to provide is the regulation of glutamate. Glutamate is a neurotransmitter in the brain that can become overstimulated. This overstimulation can lead to nerve damage.

Cons

One of the biggest complaints of those following the keto diet is the "Keto flu." You may feel weak, nauseous, suffer from a mild fever, or have body aches. These symptoms can last for a few days or up to two weeks.

The keto diet also gets a lot of criticism because of its encouragement of eating high amounts of saturated fats. Consuming too many saturated fats can put you at greater risk for heart disease and will increase bad cholesterol levels in the body.

It also emphasizes consuming excess protein, which can cause problems with the kidneys. The kidneys are responsible for metabolizing protein; on the keto diet it is recommended you consume more than the dietary recommendations. This can cause the kidneys to become overworked.

There is also more strain on the liver. Those with pre-existing liver conditions should not start a keto diet. On the keto diet, the liver puts in extra work transferring fat to fuel and if you already have a liver condition this can make your symptoms much worse.

Ketoacidosis is a serious condition that can occur from the liver over producing ketones in the body. When there is a seriously high level of ketones in the body, the blood becomes acidic and toxic. Though this condition is more common among those who have diabetes, it can occur in non-diabetics as well and may be life-threatening.

While following this plan, you will not consume a wide variety of fruits or vegetables. These food groups provide us with crucial vitamins and minerals but by excluding many of these foods you put yourself at risk for nutrient deficiencies.

Cutting out fruits, vegetables, and grains means you may not get sufficient fiber. Not getting enough fiber can cause digestive issues like constipation.

The extreme restriction of carb intake can cause cognitive function to slow. It is not uncommon for many on a keto diet to experience some form of brain impairment such as confusion or irritability.

Getting Started

Transition slowly. Cutting out carbs and sugars can be a huge shock to your system and can make it harder for you to stick with a keto diet.

While you may be eager to experience the benefits of ketosis you want to give yourself adequate time to adjust to your new eating habits. Some people may be able to adapt quickly to these changes and be successful, though most people need to take a slow and steady approach. Gradually cut out foods one at a time and replace them with keto-friendly options. Swap out your sugar-filled drinks for water. Replace your pasta with vegetables like zucchini. Use vegetables as a bread substitute—portobello mushrooms caps make great burger buns and large lettuce leaves can be used as wraps.

Be mindful of your protein consumption. Eating too much protein can delay the ketosis process or take you out of ketosis. Also be careful of your fats. It is important to be mindful of what types of fat you are eating. Some people who stick to a keto diet consume a significant amount of saturated fats which has been shown to cause serious health problems. While bacon, sausages, butter, and burgers are allowed on the keto diet, you should choose foods that have unsaturated fats instead such as:

- avocado
- olive oil
- fatty fish (salmon, tuna, sardines)
- chia seed
- flaxseed
- nuts and nut butter
- Full-fat Greek yogurt
- whole eggs

When you are starting out, keep your meals simple. Choose a lean protein, low-carb vegetables like broccoli, bell peppers, and spinach, and add in a healthy fat. Following this structure for your meals will help you transition to a keto diet with ease and put you in ketosis sooner.

Additional tips to consider:
- Be sure to get enough fiber from whole foods like vegetables and seeds.

- Drink plenty of water. When you are feeling hungry, always reach for water first as the body doesn't distinguish between thirst and hunger cues. Many people may feel hungry when instead they just need to rehydrate.
- Be mindful of your portions. Though you do not have to follow a specific portion guideline it is possible for you to overeat certain foods—like fats—and end up gaining weight.
- Be sure to get enough electrolytes. If you notice you are getting more headaches than usual when starting a keto diet this may be due to an imbalance of electrolytes. Eating bananas, avocados, and watermelon or drinking coconut water are natural ways you can replenish your electrolytes.
- Remove temptations from your home and office.
- Plan your meals and always have a keto-friendly snack on hand.

7-Day Meal Plan

Monday

Breakfast: Two eggs with spinach, onions, mushrooms, and tomatoes.

Lunch: Roasted chicken over mixed greens with feta and olives, drizzled with vinaigrette.

Dinner: Baked salmon with roasted asparagus and cauliflower mash.

Snack: Chocolate chia pudding topped with coconut and blueberries.

Tuesday

Breakfast: Tomato, basil, and spinach omelet.

Lunch: Taco salad made with ground beef or turkey over lettuce with salsa and avocado.

Dinner: Baked pork chops with broccoli and a mixed green salad.

Snack: Chocolate Peanut Butter Smoothie (blend together 1 cup of almond milk, 1 cup of spinach, 1 tablespoon of nut butter, and 1 teaspoon of cocoa powder).

Wednesday

Breakfast: Greek yogurt topped with fresh berries.

Lunch: Grilled shrimp over mixed greens with sliced avocado, drizzled with olive oil and fresh lime juice.

Dinner: Cauliflower steaks with mixed vegetables.

Snack: Kale chips and macadamia nuts.

Thursday

Breakfast: Onion and bell pepper omelet topped with avocado and salsa.

Lunch: Lettuce wraps (ground beef or turkey, bell pepper, tomatoes, and cucumber wrapped in a large lettuce leaf).

Dinner: Chicken breast stuffed with spinach and cream cheese and a side of grilled zucchini.

Snack: Raw veggie sticks with hummus.

Friday

Breakfast: Egg white muffins (made with tomato, feta, spinach, and onions).

Lunch: Stuffed portobello mushrooms (layer with tomato slices, basil, mozzarella, ground turkey or beef, and top with pesto).

Dinner: Sesame chicken and broccoli with zucchini noodles.

Snack: Salsa with parmesan chips.

Saturday

Breakfast: Hard boiled eggs, spinach, and tomatoes.

Lunch: Tofu with cauliflower rice, broccoli, and homemade peanut sauce.

Dinner: Roasted salmon stuffed with spinach, bell peppers, and ricotta. Served with roasted brussel sprouts or asparagus.

Snack: Sunflower seeds and kale chips.

Sunday

Breakfast: Baked eggs in avocado cups. To make an avocado cup simply cut an avocado in half and remove the seed. Crack the egg where the seed was and bake **at 425°F until the egg is done to your preference.**

Lunch: Roasted turkey, tomato, and avocado wrapped in lettuce leaves.

Dinner: Spaghetti squash Bolognese.

Snack: Green Smoothie (1 cup of almond milk, 1 cup of spinach, ½ an avocado, and 1 tablespoon of almond butter).

Chapter 9:

Low-Carb Diet

Carbs are often shunned because many have the misconception that all carbs are bad. The body relies on carbohydrates for essential fuel, but not all carbs are the same and the body does not distinguish between which ones energize it more efficiently. Most people are unaware that the body processes certain carbs differently. Low-carb diets have been a huge craze because there is not enough discussion on the difference between complex carbs and simple carbs. Complex carbs are digested and processed by the body slowly so that there is a constant reliable stream of fuel being supplied to it. Simple carbs are digested quickly and may cause us to have short bursts of energy followed by a major midday crash. A low-carb diet focuses on eliminating simple carbs while consuming more complex carbohydrates to supply the body with consistent energy. This chapter will teach you the best way to adopt a low-carb diet and its benefits for weight loss and beyond.

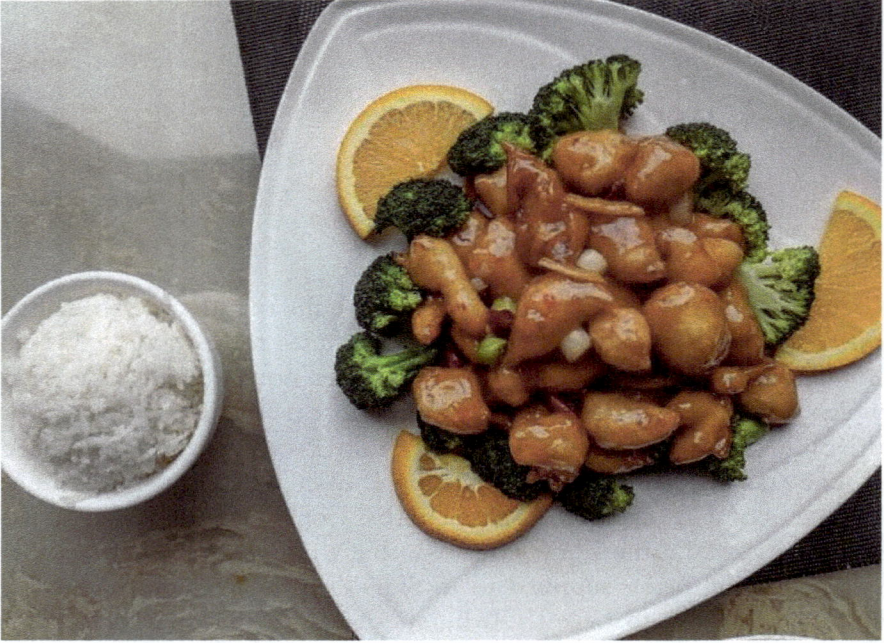

What Is a Low-Carb Diet?

A low-carb diet is a plan that reduces carbohydrate intake. The Atkins diet and Ketogenic diet are two types of low-carb diets, but they limit carb intake significantly more than a standard low-carb diet which gives you more flexibility while still limiting:

- grains
- legumes
- fruits
- bread
- sweets
- pasta
- starchy vegetables
- sugar
- milk and dairy

On a standard low-carb diet proteins and fat will make up a majority of your diet. Carbs should make up no more than 45% of your diet or no more than 900 calories of your total calorie intake if you are following a diet of 2,000 calories a day.

Keep in mind that a standard low-carb diet does emphasize consuming healthy carbs, fats, and proteins. Unlike the Keto diet, you are encouraged to eat healthy fats like avocados and olive oil over unhealthy fats. You are also encouraged to eat lean proteins and fish.

Benefits

The benefits you will experience with the Atkins diet or Keto diet are similar to those of a low-carb diet. You may not see significant improvements or differences as the other two diets cut back carb intake significantly, but you will still see noticeable changes when you go low-carb. The main thing to consider when looking over these benefits is how possible it is for you to maintain the diet long-term. A simple low-carb diet can be a great alternative for those who do not feel they can or want to restrict their carb intake significantly, but still reduce carbs to experience the benefits.

Weight Loss

There are many reasons why a low-carb diet helps you lose weight. Cutting unnecessary carbs like those from processed and sugary foods automatically helps you lose weight. Eating a diet higher in fat and protein helps you feel fuller for longer so you eat fewer calories naturally. You will see rapid weight loss when you first start a low-carb diet which helps motivate you to stick with it.

You Lose More Visceral Fat

Visceral fat is harmful as it is stored fat that builds up around the organs, typically in the abdomen area. This fat is associated with an increased risk of inflammation, insulin resistance, metabolic dysfunction, heart disease, and type 2 diabetes. A low-carb diet helps eliminate this harmful fat as it causes the body to use it for fuel when there's limited carbs.

Other Advantages

As with any other low-carb diet it is possible to experience a wide range of benefits. If a low-carb diet is approached properly, where you focus on consuming complex carbs while eliminating simple carbs, you can see significant improvements to your health. Some additional benefits of a low-carb diet include:

- Lower levels of triglycerides (bad cholesterol).
- Lower blood sugar levels.
- Managing insulin levels.
- Helping manage metabolic syndrome.
- Improving brain health.

Cons

Low-carb diets have shown to be highly effective for weight loss and improved health in the short-term. While these short-term benefits are great, they need to be weighed against the long term problems that can arise. For many, sticking to a low-carb diet can cause serious health risks like an increased risk of cardiovascular disease.

You may suffer from digestive issues like constipation. A low-carb diet can be low in fiber which is essential for digestion. When you remove things like whole grains and certain fruits from your diet, you are limiting the amount of fiber you will consume as these foods are rich sources of fiber.

If your low-carb diet is also a high-fat diet you may be putting yourself at greater risk for cardiovascular disease. Most people who switch to low-carb skip eating nutritious vegetables that are beneficial to their health and choose to fill up on high-fat foods like burgers, bacon, and steaks. These foods can raise LDL (bad) cholesterol. Bad cholesterol blocks the arteries and puts you at greater risk for serious health problems. Also, these high-fat foods increase homocysteine levels which is an amino acid shown to increase one's risk of heart disease (Torres, 2020).

There is also an increased risk of kidney stones. Kidney stones can be extremely painful and could block fluids from exiting the body. If stones cause this fluid to remain stagnant, bacteria will build up in the body and lead to a kidney infection. Kidney stones are predominantly caused by dehydration but another common cause is uric acid. Animal protein and fish break down and turn into uric acid. Consuming a diet high in animal protein results in excess acid in the body which causes kidney stones to form. Additionally, consuming high amounts of animal protein reduces citrate in the body which is necessary to prevent the formation of kidney stones. Since a low-carb diet promotes increasing the amount of animal protein you consume, you will be putting yourself at greater risk for developing these painful stones.

Getting Started

Track what you eat. Many people do not realize how many unnecessary carbs and junk foods they eat throughout the day. Spend two weeks keeping a food journal to see what you are eating and when. Write everything you eat and drink in the journal honestly. If you don't include those fries you swipe from your kid's plate, you will not accurately know what you are eating and these little habits can add up to major weight gain. Once you know what you are eating, how much, and when, you can create a more effective plan to go low-carb.

Stick with lean proteins. Protein-rich foods help curb appetite so you will feel fuller for longer periods of time.

Begin by cutting the unhealthy carbs. The main benefit of a low-carb diet is not necessarily the fact that you are cutting carbs but instead because you are cutting out processed carbs. Swap your unhealthy snacks like chips and sweets with fruit, vegetables, and nuts.

Cut back on sweet drinks. Soda, juices, and specialty coffees contain high amounts of sugar. Many people who go on a low-carb diet neglect how many calories and sugar they consume through their drinks.

Consider an induction phase where for two weeks you significantly cut back on your carbohydrate intake. Reducing carb intake to 20 or 30 grams a day can help you jumpstart your weight loss and help eliminate food cravings. After these two weeks you can begin to add in more carbs throughout the day but keep it on the lower side to about 100 grams a day.

Do not cut out all carbs. Carbs are beneficial and your body does need the nutrients and fuel that carbohydrates provide. Instead of trying to cut out all carbs, stick with whole grains and fresh fruit that will provide you with essential vitamins and minerals. You can still limit how much of these you eat but be mindful to eat more wholesome carbs over processed ones.

7-Day Meal Plan

Monday

Breakfast: Breakfast burrito (two eggs, bacon, tomatoes, onions, and a bell pepper, wrapped in a whole wheat tortilla).

Lunch: Avocado salad over mixed greens and two tablespoons of vinaigrette dressing.

Snack: An orange.

Dinner: Shrimp scampi with zucchini noodles.

Snack: ½ cup of fresh raspberries.

Tuesday

Breakfast: Steel-cut oats with blueberries and raspberries.

Lunch: Cauliflower rice bowl (add in some tomatoes, zucchini, carrots, or bell peppers).

Snack: Two plums.

Dinner: Pork chops with garlic-roasted broccoli and cauliflower.

Snack: ½ cup of fresh fruit with Greek yogurt.

Wednesday

Breakfast: Two eggs with sausage and a banana.

Lunch: Tuna salad over mixed greens and an orange.

Snack: 12 almonds.

Dinner: Roasted chicken with spaghetti squash and tomato sauce.

Snack: A cup of grapes and an ounce of cheddar cheese.

Thursday

Breakfast: Superfood Smoothie (blend together 1 cup of almond milk, ½ cup spinach, ½ cup kale, ½ cup blueberries, ½ cup strawberries, and ice to thicken).

Lunch: Zucchini noodles with turkey bolognese.

Snack: An apple.

Dinner: Grilled salmon with sautéed spinach and roasted potatoes.

Snack: ½ cup of raspberries and 8 almonds.

Friday

Breakfast: A cup of fresh berries topped with ½ cup of greek yogurt, 1 teaspoon of chia seeds, and 1 tablespoon of shredded unsweetened coconut.

Lunch: Egg salad wrapped in lettuce.

Snack: An orange and 8 almonds.

Dinner: Cauliflower mac and cheese (you may add in peas and chopped bacon).

Snack: An apple an ounce of cheese.

Saturday

Breakfast: Spinach, cheese, and tomato omelet with turkey bacon.

Lunch: Zucchini boats filled with ground turkey, cheddar, cheese, bell pepper, onions, and tomatoes.

Snack: Avocado Smoothie (1 avocado, 1 pear, 2 tablespoons cacao powder, and 1 cup of almond milk).

Dinner: Vegetable soup.

Snack: Fresh berries topped with greek yogurt and almond slivers.

Sunday

Breakfast: Low-carb blueberry muffins.

Lunch: Chicken salad wrap with lettuce.

Snack: Two hard-boiled eggs and an orange.

Dinner: Beef stroganoff with a side salad topped with a citrus vinaigrette.

Snack: A pear and an ounce of cheddar cheese.

Chapter 10:

Mayo Clinic Diet

The Mayo Clinic diet is a life-long solution to losing weight and maintaining it. This diet is not just about what you eat. This diet focuses on a wide range of things that contribute to a healthy lifestyle including exercise, sleep, and stress management. Each of these areas has a tendency to influence our eating habits and by addressing these matters it allows us to take full control over our health and weight.

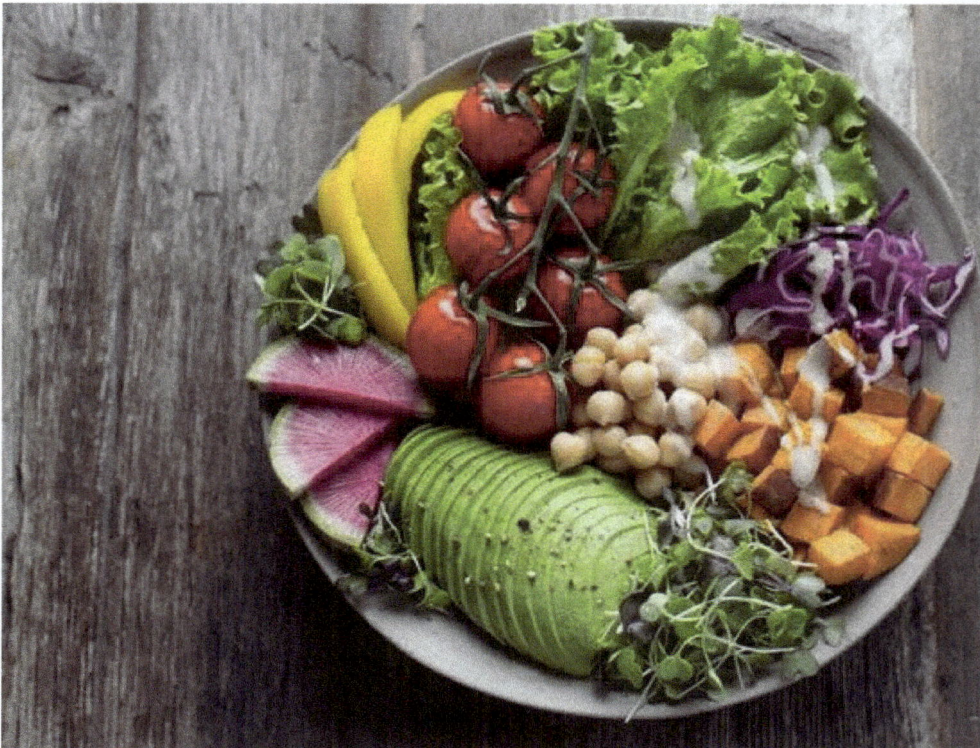

What Is the Mayo Clinic Diet?

Unlike most diets that simply restrict foods, this diet emphasizes changing eating habits. The diet consists of two phases where you learn to rethink when, what, and how you eat while incorporating additional habits for better health.

Phase one is the "lost it" phase. During this phase you focus on adopting five healthy habits, eliminating five unhealthy habits, and adding in five bonus habits. The bonus habits are not essential but are encouraged to help you stay committed and make life-long changes. In the first phase, you will cut out all sugary foods and drinks. Other bad habits can include:

- Avoid snacking with the exception of fruits and vegetables.
- Stop eating processed meats.
- Eliminate processed flour and grains.
- Don't eat when you're bored.
- Don't eat while watching television

Some good habits to adopt may include:
- Drink more water.
- Eat more fruits and vegetables.
- Have one or two meatless days.
- Eat more fish.
- Make more home-cooked meals.
- Pack your lunch
- Switch from full fat to low-fat dairy.
- Start the day with a healthy breakfast.

There are also bonus habits you can add during this first phase such as:
- Keeping journals to track food, activity levels, or daily goals.
- Exercising for one hour a day.
- Eat your vegetables first
- Limit screen time.
- Practice mindfulness when eating.

- Listen to your body: When you are hungry eat fresh fruit or a handful of nuts as a snack. When you are full stop eating; you do not have to clear your plate.

The "lose it" phase lasts for two weeks and is geared to prepare you for the "live it" phase.

During phase two, you are transitioning to healthier lifestyle habits. You will gain a deeper understanding of portion size, meal planning, how many calories to eat, and how to make better food choices. You also will incorporate habits like exercising and stress management for better overall health.

The Mayo Clinic Diet also utilizes a pyramid to help create a balanced healthy diet.

- The base of the pyramid represents fruits and vegetables. In this tier, you can eat as much as you want without restrictions.
- The next tier represents whole grains. This tier includes items like quinoa, brown rice, oats, and whole wheat bread. This tier should be consumed in moderation.
- Above the whole grain tier comes protein. Proteins should come from lean meats, legumes, fish, and some low-fat dairy. Make sure to consume proteins in moderation and do not eat more protein than whole grains.
- The fourth tier is made up of healthy fats. This tier includes nuts, olive oil, and avocados. Healthy fats make up a small portion of your diet. As a general rule, you want to consume less fat than you do proteins.
- At the top of the pyramid is the smallest tier—the sweets. This tier should only be consumed occasionally; no more than 75 calories a day should come from sweets. This tier is also only added during the second phase of the diet.

Benefits

The Mayo Clinic diet does more than address what you eat. Since it focuses on confronting eating habits, there are many more benefits you can experience from this diet. These additional benefits may make the Mayo Clinic diet a lifestyle choice.

Weight Loss

There are several reasons why the Mayo Clinic diet promotes weight loss. This diet consists of eating more whole foods (fruits, vegetables, and whole grains). Replacing the foods that cause you to gain weight with whole foods will naturally trigger weight loss. The diet also recommends eating foods high in fiber which help to suppress appetite by keeping you feeling full for longer. The diet also suggests getting moderate exercise daily. Adding exercise along with eating a healthier diet is a more effective way to lose weight than just changing your diet alone. Exercising helps build muscle mass. Since muscle requires more energy it burns more calories. Even while you are resting your muscles are using calories. If the body requires more fuel because of the extra energy the muscles are using, it converts stored fat to be dispersed to the cells for energy. If you incorporate weight training or weight resistance exercises into your routine you can speed up this process.

Restrict Calories Without Calorie Counting

This diet does not require you to count calories but you will naturally lower your calorie consumption by consuming more whole foods. The Mayo Clinic diet is designed to promote a calorie deficiency of 500 to 1,000 calories a day (during the second phase). This reduction in calories will result in losing one to two pounds a week. While this seems like you will not be losing much, it is an effective approach to managing your weight long-term. Each of those pounds will add up and in no time you could lose 15, 25, or 40 pounds.

Life-Long Eating Plan

The Mayo Clinic diet emphasizes behavior-based changes to promote weight loss. Focusing on changing eating behaviors as opposed to finding temporary solutions will lead to life-long changes. Changing eating behaviors includes when and why you eat, mindlessly eating while watching television, or feeding your emotions. Recognizing these eating habits and changing them will result in keeping weight off and improve your health long-term.

Well-Researched Dieting Approach

This plan was created by multiple medical professionals. The diet takes into account various studies that outline the best ways to lose weight, optimize health, and simplify weight management for life. Multiple studies show that a diet rich in fruits and vegetables reduces the risk of health conditions like heart disease and diabetes (Groves, 2019).

Easy to Follow

Aside from the first two weeks, this diet plan does not implement major restrictions. Instead, it places a major focus on replacing unwanted habits with better-for-you habits. It helps you identify when you may overeat, what foods you are most tempted by, and lets you create an effective plan to combat these and put an end to your unhealthy diet habits.

What makes this diet unique is that it doesn't just focus on eating habits. You will learn how to portion your foods and the best foods to eat for optimal health but the Mayo Clinic diet also encourages additional healthy habits into its plan. When you begin to make beneficial changes to more than just what you eat, you not only improve your health, but you will find your quality of life improves.

Cons

The "lose it" phase, though only two weeks, can be a challenge to follow. No sugar, no eating out, and incorporating exercise into your day is a lot to start all at once. All these new healthy lifestyle changes can be overwhelming to anyone and may be difficult to commit to in the beginning.

The emphasis on planning, prepping, and cooking your own meals can be more time-consuming than many have the time for. If you are looking for a diet plan that has prepared meals, made for you meal plans, or meal kits to make preparing meals easier, you are not going to find it with this diet. Learning how to plan and make your own meals is part of this diet's process to ensure you can make the necessary lifestyle changes to stick with this way of eating for the long-term.

You also need to rely on more self-motivation. You must want to make a lifelong change to stick with and incorporate the necessary healthy habits. Many people start a diet for the sole purpose of losing weight. Once they lose the weight they go back to how they used to eat because most diets are not meant to be adhered to for life. Losing weight and keeping it off requires commitment to this way of eating. It needs to be something you can make into a lifestyle choice.

What makes motivating yourself harder is that it can be hard to find the right information to help you along the way. There are plenty of articles about this diet available online, but many are contradictory and confusing. To fully understand how to get through the first phase and successfully transition into the second phase it is encouraged that you purchase *The Mayo Clinic Diet* book which provides step-by-step instructions. The book can be useful but is another expense and you need to make time to read through the whole thing.

There is also the struggle many face when they try to incorporate exercise into their dieting plan. Finding time to get in a consecutive 30 minutes of physical activity is too much to ask for those who already have hectic schedules. While exercise is essential for living a healthy life and helps reduce the risk of chronic health conditions, most people do not like to exercise. You won't see rapid weight loss or improve your health if you skip on incorporating exercise along with your diet changes.

Getting Started

Schedule workout times or take note of when you can add in more physical activity to your day. You do not have to get all your exercise done in one shot. You can break up your exercise times by walking for 10 minutes three times a day. Get in two 15-minute cardio sessions. Do 15 minutes of running in the morning and 15 minutes of weight lifting after work. Find an exercise routine that fits with your schedule. If you can get 30 minutes in all at once, stick with that. If you find you keep skipping exercise because you don't have time, break the time up and fit it in where you can.

Understand what your caloric intake should be. You do not need to count calories to lose weight. A basic understanding of how many calories your body needs to feel energized throughout the day is all you need to know. Women should consume between 1,200 to 1,600 calories a day while men should consume 1,400 to 1,800 calories a day.

A 1,400 caloric intake breaks down to:

- four or more servings of fruits and vegetables a day
- five servings of carbs
- four servings of protein or dairy
- three servings of fat

7-Day Meal Plan

Monday

Breakfast: 1 cup whole-grain cereal with low-fat or almond milk, topped with ½ cup of fresh berries.

Lunch: Grilled chicken salad (grilled chicken, mixed greens, tomatoes, bell pepper, green onion, and grape halves, drizzled with extra virgin olive oil and two tablespoons of red wine vinegar).

Dinner: Three ounces of lemon basil grilled tuna, ½ cup of brown rice and 1 cup of steamed zucchini or yellow summer squash.

Snack: Carrot and celery sticks with a tablespoon of nut butter.

Tuesday

Breakfast: A cup of oats made with nonfat milk topped with banana slices and a cup of fresh strawberries.

Lunch: Tuna salad with a sliced bell pepper in a pita and an apple.

Dinner: Red curry lentil and kale soup.

Snack: Eight almonds and a cup of grapes.

Wednesday

Breakfast: Two hard-boiled eggs with two slices of whole-wheat toast and avocado slices.

Lunch: Quinoa bowl (with sweet potatoes, sautéed spinach, bell peppers, and mushrooms) tossed in a lime dressing.

Dinner: Grilled pork tenderloin with a balsamic reduction. Served with mixed greens and sautéed green beans topped with almonds.

Snack: A pear and ¾ cup blueberries.

Thursday

Breakfast: Baked Apple cinnamon oats.

Lunch: Strawberry and spinach salad with grilled chicken.

Dinner: Grilled shrimp skewers with a half cup of brown rice and grilled vegetables.

Snack: A banana and six whole-wheat crackers.

Friday

Breakfast: Greek yogurt with kiwi, blueberries, raspberries and homemade granola.

Lunch: Black bean wraps.

Dinner: Roasted chicken with sweet potatoes, brussel sprouts, and beets.

Snack: Bell pepper sticks with two tablespoons of hummus.

Saturday

Breakfast: Half a grapefruit, two hard-boiled eggs, and a slice of whole-wheat toast.

Lunch: Mediterranean chopped salad (tomatoes, cucumbers, onions, red bell pepper, spinach, parsley, chickpeas, and olives). Drizzle with extra virgin olive oil and red wine vinegar or lemon juice.

Dinner: Turkey meatloaf with cauliflower mash and mixed greens.

Snack: Grilled apples and peaches.

Sunday

Breakfast: Vegetable omelet and half a grapefruit.

Lunch: Black beans with a mixed green salad and roasted sweet potato fries.

Dinner: Roasted squash soup.

Snack: Roasted chickpeas and a cup of melon.

Chapter 11:

Mediterranean Diet

The Mediterranean diet is a whole-foods plant-based eating plan. It is considered a semi-vegetarian diet that puts an emphasis on eating more fish and seafood over red meat and poultry. The Mediterranean diet was created after much research was conducted on individuals living around the Mediterranean Sea. These individuals were shown to have the best health when compared to other people from around the world. The idea of this diet is not just to replicate what people ate in these regions but to also adopt many of their lifestyle behaviors such as walking more and make meals a time for connection.

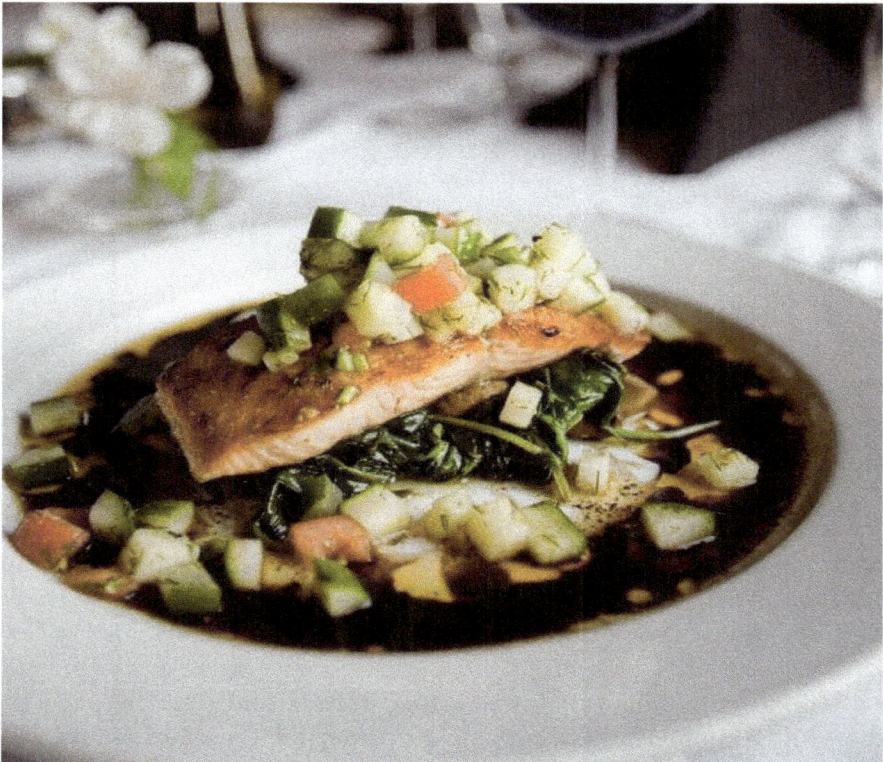

What Is the Mediterranean Diet?

The Mediterranean diet dates back to the 1950s and represents the traditional eating patterns of those living around the Mediterranean sea. It encourages eating fresh fruits, vegetables, and fish just as those living in the Mediterranean ate in the 50's. Prepackaged, processed foods, and sugary drinks are excluded, as these were not available in the Mediterranean regions. Various studies conducted on this region highlights how these foods are absent from their diet and can be credited for their better health.

The diet is straightforward and flexible as there are some variations depending on which region of the Mediterranean you look at. As a general consensus, though, the diet encourages eating plant-based whole-foods. Foods that are consumed the most on the diet include:

- fresh fruit and vegetables
- nuts and seeds
- legumes
- whole grains
- fish and seafood
- extra virgin olive oil
- herbs and spices
- eggs
- dairy

Water is essential on the diet but it also encourages consuming up to a glass of red wine a day. Coffee and tea are also allowed but you should limit any sugar or cream you may add to these.

As you will notice, red meat and poultry are not on the list. While these items are not cut out, they are consumed rarely. Many people on the Mediterranean diet limit their consumption of poultry to once a week or a few times a month. Red meat should only be consumed a few times a month or only on special occasions like birthdays, anniversaries, or holidays. Instead, fish and seafood take the place of these other animal products. You will often see meals of whole fish being shared at dinner tables or during lunchtime. Lamb is also consumed regularly on the Mediterranean diet as often as once a week.

Foods that are typically avoided on the Mediterranean diet include:

- foods and drinks with added sugar
- refined grains (white bread and pasta, chips, crackers)
- foods that contain trans fats (margarine, fried foods)
- processed foods (fast food, prepackaged meals, microwaveable meals, granola bars)
- refined oils (soybean oil, grapeseed oil, canola oil)
- processed meat

Benefits

The Mediterranean diet gives you more flexibility to choose wholesome and delicious foods. The foods that are strongly encouraged on this diet have been studied extensively to highlight their health benefits. If you have been considering a Mediterranean diet, below are some health benefits to consider.

Flexible

The Mediterranean diet does not restrict any foods so you can cater it to your preferences and lifestyle. There are some foods you might want to avoid but this diet doesn't forbid them. You have the freedom to enjoy desserts, snacks, and delicious filling meals.

Weight Loss

As with many other diets, the Mediterranean Diet limits the amount of processed foods, added sugar, refined oils, and red meat you consume. Whenever you remove these items from your diet you will experience weight loss. The Mediterranean diet also favors fruits and vegetables which tend to have fewer calories.

Improve Blood Sugar Levels

Consuming a diet of fresh fruits and vegetables has been studied extensively for its effect on blood sugar levels. The Mediterranean diet specifically has been shown to improve levels of hemoglobin A1C and lower fasting sugar levels (Sleiman et al., 2015). Hemoglobin A1C is used to show long-term blood sugar control; managing these levels indicates the body's ability to properly use the fuel it is provided in the most effective way.

Can Help Prevent and Manage Diabetes

Insulin resistance is a serious issue for those with type 2 diabetes. This condition means the body is not able to absorb the glucose in the blood which causes spikes in blood sugar levels. The Mediterranean diet has been shown to provide as much benefit as a low-carb diet in terms of improving insulin resistance (Trico et al., 2021). When you add this to the other benefits of the diet such as weight loss and improving blood sugar levels, the Mediterranean diet can help those with diabetes or at greater risk of developing the conditions to manage or prevent it.

Heart Healthy Diet

The Mediterranean diet has been compared to a variety of other diets. When compared to a low-fat diet the Mediterranean diet was more effective at slowing down the buildup of plaque in the arteries (Gunnars and Link, 2021). Plaque build up is a serious risk for developing heart disease. The other benefits the diet provides—lowering blood pressure and reducing inflammation—aids in its heart-healthy benefits. This eating plan encourages consuming hearty healthy fats while minimizing or eliminating unhealthy ones. This not only will protect your heart and keep it functioning properly, but it also prolongs your life expectancy.

Promotes a Healthy Brain

There are many reasons the Mediterranean diet can help with cognitive function and slow down age-related degeneration. The Mediterranean diet encourages the consumption of wild-caught fish, which contains a significant amount of omega-3 fatty acids. Various studies indicate that omega-3 fatty acids are essential for a healthy brain. Other studies have found that the Mediterranean diet can help lower the risk of dementia and Alzheimer's disease. Additional reviews of studies show that individuals who follow a Mediterranean diet have better attention, memory, and processing speed than those who followed other diet plans (Loughrey et al., 2017).

Encourages a Healthy Lifestyle

Along with eating more plant-based whole foods, the Mediterranean diet focuses on other aspects of an overall healthy lifestyle. It encourages getting plenty of exercise to model the daily physical activity of those living in the Mediterranean. Since most individuals in the area relied on walking or cycling as their primary mode of transportation, this is credited for better health. There is also an emphasis on sharing meals and remaining present while eating. Typical of those in the region sitting down and connecting with others while preparing and eating a meal, these eating behaviors are likely to have benefited those individuals' mental health.

Cons

The lack of calorie restriction or limit on the amount of fats and carbs you can eat can result in consuming more empty calories, which may make weight loss more difficult. The diet's flexibility leaves a lot of room to consume items that will not provide many health benefits. Many people claim to follow a Mediterranean diet but consume high amounts of processed oil or added sugar. Without clear guidelines, some people who have tried other diets may struggle to stick to a more plant-based approach with the Mediterranean diet.

This diet does not eliminate foods, which means creating a healthy eating plan is essential. You will want to ensure you are eating more nutrient-rich foods, but since nothing is off-limits it can be easier to indulge on foods that are not packed with nutrients.

If you would much rather eat a steak instead of tuna or salmon, you will not enjoy this diet. This plan encourages eating plenty of fresh fish and seafood over animal proteins.

Getting Started

Switching to a Mediterranean diet is not complex. You can start a Mediterranean diet the same way you would start a low-carb or flexitarian diet. There are a few things that make the Mediterranean diet different from others. Remember the following when you get started on a Mediterranean diet:

- Use more olive oil. Use it to cook with instead of butter or add it to dishes for more flavor (drizzle it over salmon or stir it in your mashed potatoes).
- Eat more fatty fish like salmon, mackerel, and sardines.
- Add vegetables to every meal, including snacks.
- Eat whole grains like quinoa, barley, and oats. Do not just switch to whole grain foods like whole-wheat pasta; experiment with grains in whole form.
- Carry around nuts like almonds, pecans, and Brazil nuts to snack on.
- Swap your sugar-filled dessert for fresh fruits.
- Enjoy red wine with your meal.

- Get everyone in the house on board. Make meal planning and cooking a new family activity. Have your kids help with the cooking and bond with them as they help.
- It is traditional for lunch and dinner to be served alongside whole grain or sourdough bread with olive oil and balsamic vinegar for dipping.
- You can have snacks in between meals but keep these to fresh fruits, raw veggies and hummus, or a few nuts and cheeses.

7-Day Meal Plan

Monday

Breakfast: Steel cut oats with banana and walnuts.

Lunch: Hummus, red bell pepper sticks, cucumber, carrot sticks, and onions in a whole wheat pita with a half cup of fresh raspberries and blackberries.

Dinner: Baked salmon with lemon, olive oil, potatoes, and roasted vegetables served with sourdough bread.

Dessert: Figs and mixed nuts.

Tuesday

Breakfast: Green Smoothie (1 cup of almond milk, ½ cup of Greek yogurt, 1 cup of spinach, 1 banana, ½ cup of pineapple, 1 tablespoon of chia seeds, and 1 teaspoon of pure maple syrup or organic honey).

Lunch: Vegetable chili.

Dinner: Whole grain pasta with spinach, onions, mushrooms, and broccoli with pesto.

Dessert: Chia seed pudding.

Wednesday

Breakfast: Baked oats with apples, cinnamon, and walnuts.

Lunch: Gyro served with cucumber, tomato, and onion salad (drizzle the salad with extra virgin olive oil and balsamic reduction).

Dinner: Moussaka (eggplant lasagna) with a side of mixed greens.

Dessert: Greek yogurt with pistachios, honey, and melon.

Thursday

Breakfast: Avocado toast and a fruit smoothie (blend together ½ cup of almond milk, ½ cup of greek yogurt, 1 cup of kale, ½ cup of pineapples, ¼ cup of blueberries, and two figs).

Lunch: Shrimp salad with mixed greens, tomatoes, cucumbers and sliced yellow bell pepper drizzled with a citrus vinaigrette.

Dinner: Falafel with steamed green beans, mixed green salad, and a whole grain pita served with hummus, tahini sauce, and tzatziki.

Dessert: Cottage cheese with sliced peaches and pineapple.

Friday

Breakfast: Blueberry overnight oats.

Lunch: Tuna, roasted vegetables, and quinoa salad.

Dinner: Spaghetti squash lasagna.

Dessert: Apple slices with nut butter.

Saturday

Breakfast: Fresh crepes and mixed berries drizzled with pure maple syrup or honey.

Lunch: Lentil soup.

Dinner: Grilled tuna steaks with spinach salad, couscous, and cauliflower mash.

Dessert: Raspberry sorbet.

Sunday

Breakfast: Scrambled eggs with skillet potatoes (cook potatoes in olive oil with green peppers, onions, and herbs) and a slice of whole-grain bread with a plum or an orange.

Lunch: Raw veggies with hummus, pita bread, and fresh fruit salad.

Dinner: Lamb chops with roasted potatoes, brussel sprouts, and broccoli. Serve with a side of mixed green salad.

Dessert: Greek yogurt with blueberries and honey.

Chapter 12:

MIND Diet

Mediterranean-DASH Intervention for Neurodegenerative Delay or MIND diet focuses on brain health. As you get older, brain health becomes more important as age-related cognitive decline may start becoming a concern. This diet combines benefits from both the Mediterranean diet and the Dash diet. While the focus is on improving brain health you will learn in this chapter that the MIND diet can help you lose weight and feel great.

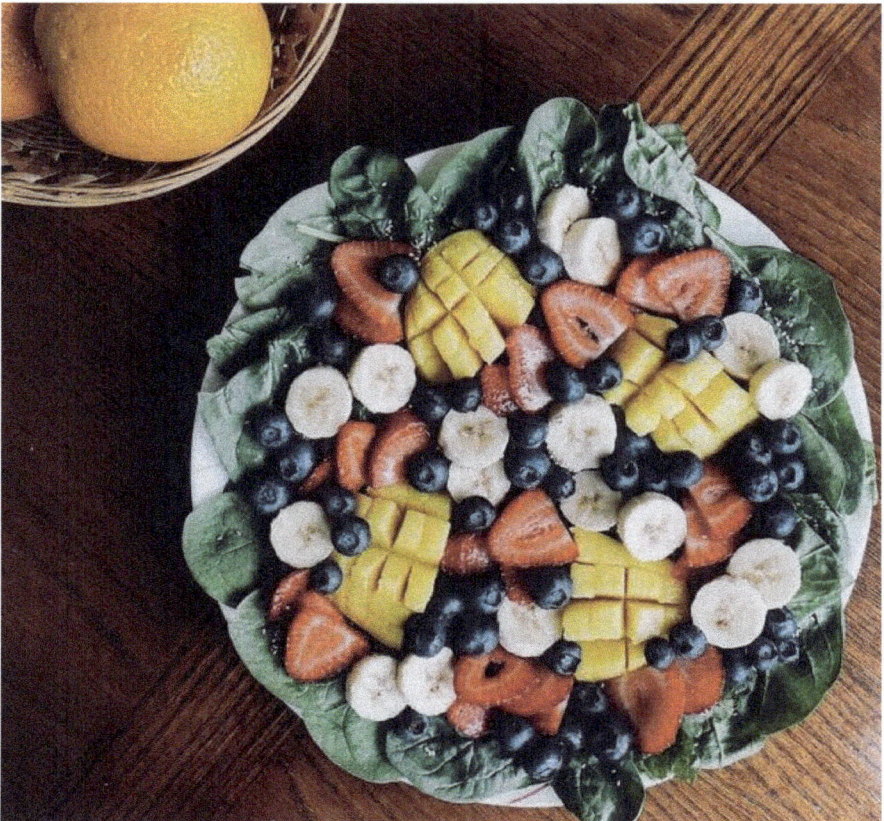

What Is the MIND Diet?

The MIND diet is a hybrid of the Mediterranean diet and the DASH diet. This diet focuses on plant-based food sources and portion control. It recommends eating more brain-healthy foods such as:

- leafy greens
- blueberries
- strawberries
- olive oil
- beans

These foods provide a mix of brain-boosting benefits such as antioxidants and anti-inflammatory properties. They also help lower beta-amyloid plaque which builds up in the brain and causes nerve damage. A high deposit of this plaque can cause memory problems and serious cognitive decline which often leads to dementia.

The MIND diet typically promotes consuming unprocessed or minimally processed foods. Animal-based foods, high saturated fats, and added sugars are limited. As a general guideline, there are 10 food groups encouraged on the MIND diet. These foods and their recommended portions include:

- whole grains: three servings a day
- fruits: at least one serving, plus a minimum of two servings of berries (as snacks) per day.
- leafy greens: at least one serving a day
- other vegetables: two servings a day (not including leafy greens)
- beans and legumes: at least four servings a week or every other day
- poultry: two serving a week
- fish: at least two servings a week
- nuts (as snacks): once a day or at least five servings a week.
- olive oil: daily use
- meat and dairy: sparingly, no more than four times a week.

The diet also encourages having a glass of red wine every day for its antioxidant benefits. The only exception to this glass-a-day recommendation is for those who have been diagnosed with Parkinson's disease. Parkinson's can cause individuals to have balance issues; having a glass of wine could make this symptom worse and result in injury.

Food items you will want to limit to one serving a week include:

- butter and margarine and other saturated or trans fats (no more than a tablespoon a day)
- cheese
- red meats
- fish high in mercury (mackerel, swordfish, ahi tuna)
- fried foods
- sweets, desserts, and pastries

Benefits

Though you will learn that there are many brain-boosting benefits to the MIND diet, there are additional factors you should consider. If you are at greater risk for certain cognitive conditions, the MIND diet might be high on your list of things to try. If you are older and are experiencing more moments of brain fog, the MIND diet can help you gain mental clarity. Below you will learn the many ways the MIND diet can benefit your brain and overall health.

Though the MIND diet does not focus on weight loss, making the recommended diet changes do promote weight loss. When you make these dietary changes long-term, there are plenty of health benefits you will experience.

Protects Against Alzheimer's

Various studies have been conducted to understand the connection between what we eat and brain health. Through these studies, it has been found that certain foods can cause one to be at a higher risk for cognitive decline like Alzheimer's. One such study published in *Alzheimer's and Dementia* tracked over 900 participants' diets for four and a half years. Those taking part in the study were between the ages of 58 and 98. Participants stuck with either a Mediterranean diet, DASH diet, or MIND diet. The results showed that individuals who ate according to the MIND diet lowered their risk of developing Alzheimer's by over 50% (Morris et al., 2015). Those who followed the MIND diet for the longest period of time saw the greatest reduction of risk for developing Alzheimer's.

Improve Brain Health

The MIND diet focuses on improving all functions of the brain. By consuming more antioxidant-rich foods and anti-inflammatory foods, you are eliminating many free radicals in the body. These free radicals build up over time and can accumulate as oxidative stress in the brain, which is a plaque that slows down cognition. The mind diet also focuses on eating nutrient-dense foods; specifically those rich in B vitamins, iron, zinc, and omega-3. These nutrients strengthen and support neurotransmitters that carry messages to and from the brain. Keeping these transmitters functioning optimally results in a better mood, sleep, concentration, and overall improved bodily functions.

Protects the Brain Against Age-Related Conditions

Several studies highlight how the MIND diet can slow the aging process of the brain by over seven years (Morris et al., 2015). On the MIND diet you are encouraged to incorporate plenty of leafy greens. These vegetables contain powerful nutrients for brain health such as vitamin E, folate, flavonoids, and carotenoids. These nutrients help promote brain cell growth and keep neurotransmitters functioning properly Eating blueberries and strawberries as a snack provides flavonoids that have been shown to help slow down the rate of cognitive decline.

Easy to Follow

You do not need to track calories on the MIND diet, which makes it less overwhelming and easier to follow for most. As with most other healthy diets, the main focus is on increasing your consumption of vegetables while cutting back on processed foods.

Cons

The guidelines for the MIND diet are relaxed which can result in slacking off more with proper nutrition and exercise. Studies have shown that even if you follow the diet partially, you can still experience many of the cognitive benefits. While this sounds like an ideal way to improve your health, it also sets you up to slack off more than you should. With this flexibility, it can also result in counter-production. You may follow some of the diet suggestions and then give yourself a free pass to over-consuming foods that can cause poor brain health.

While the MIND diet can help protect and improve some cognitive functions, diet alone can not control all factors that lead to cognitive decline. Some individuals are genetically predisposed to be at greater risk of certain brain disorders and conditions. The MIND diet cannot eliminate all risks for developing certain mental conditions.

Getting Started

You can utilize any of the tips from the Mediterranean diet and DASH diet. A few other tips that can help you transition to the MIND diet quickly include:

- Add in more colorful vegetables and fruits.
- Replace processed or refined grains with whole grains.
- Begin to cut back on red meats or replace these items with fatty fish or poultry.

- Cut out sugary beverages.
- Swap sweet treats for fresh berries.
- When shopping, stick to the perimeter of the store. The outside aisle is where you will find fresh produce, seafood, and other foods you want to stock up on with this diet.

7-Day Meal Plan

Monday

Breakfast: Vegetable omelet with a slice of whole grain toast.

Lunch: Lentil, avocado, and arugula salad topped with a citrus Greek yogurt dressing.

Dinner: Ground turkey and quinoa chili.

Snack: Banana Strawberry Smoothie (blend together one cup almond milk, a frozen banana, and a cup of strawberries).

Tuesday

Breakfast: Blueberry walnut whole-wheat pancakes.

Lunch: Kale Caesar salad.

Dinner: Grilled chicken with black beans, roasted radish, and asparagus.

Snack: Whole-wheat toast with nut butter and a banana.

Wednesday

Breakfast: Greek yogurt with fresh berries and almonds.

Lunch: Cucumber, red bell pepper, carrot, and celery with hummus wrapped in a whole grain tortilla and a half cup of grapes or melon on the side.

Dinner: Whole-grain pasta primavera.

Snack: Zucchini and kale chips.

Thursday

Breakfast: Oatmeal with fresh blueberries and walnuts.

Lunch: Tuna salad sandwich on whole-wheat bread.

Dinner: Baked salmon with roasted broccoli and a side salad.

Snack: Green Smoothie (blend together 1 cup of almond milk, ½ an avocado, 1 cup of kale, ½ cup of pineapple, and ½ cup of strawberries).

Friday

Breakfast: Scrambled egg, tomato, and avocado on a whole-wheat bagel with a banana.

Lunch: Spinach salad with strawberries, chickpeas, and almonds with an olive oil dressing.

Dinner: Honey Dijon roasted chicken with steamed green beans and a baked potato.

Snack: Apple slices and nut butter.

Saturday

Breakfast: Spinach and mushroom omelet.

Lunch: Turkey with tomato, lettuce, and hummus on whole-wheat bread, with a side of carrot sticks or baby carrots.

Dinner: Chicken and vegetable stir-fry.

Snack: Chocolate chia seed pudding.

Sunday

Breakfast: Overnight oats with strawberries.

Lunch: Chicken gyro with tomatoes, onions, and cucumber on a whole wheat pita.

Dinner: Carrot and ginger soup with a whole-wheat roll.

Snack: Grapes and sunflower seeds.

Chapter 13:

Paleo Diet

Were our ancestors healthy? Many people think that the way our ancestors hunted and gathered and were constantly on the move resulted in them being in prime physical shape. This belief in the way we lived hundreds of years ago sparked a trend in the way some people eat. The Paleo diet was crafted to mimic the eating habits of our ancient ancestors. For some, this way of eating simplifies meal planning and prep while others struggle to let go of our modern food convenience.

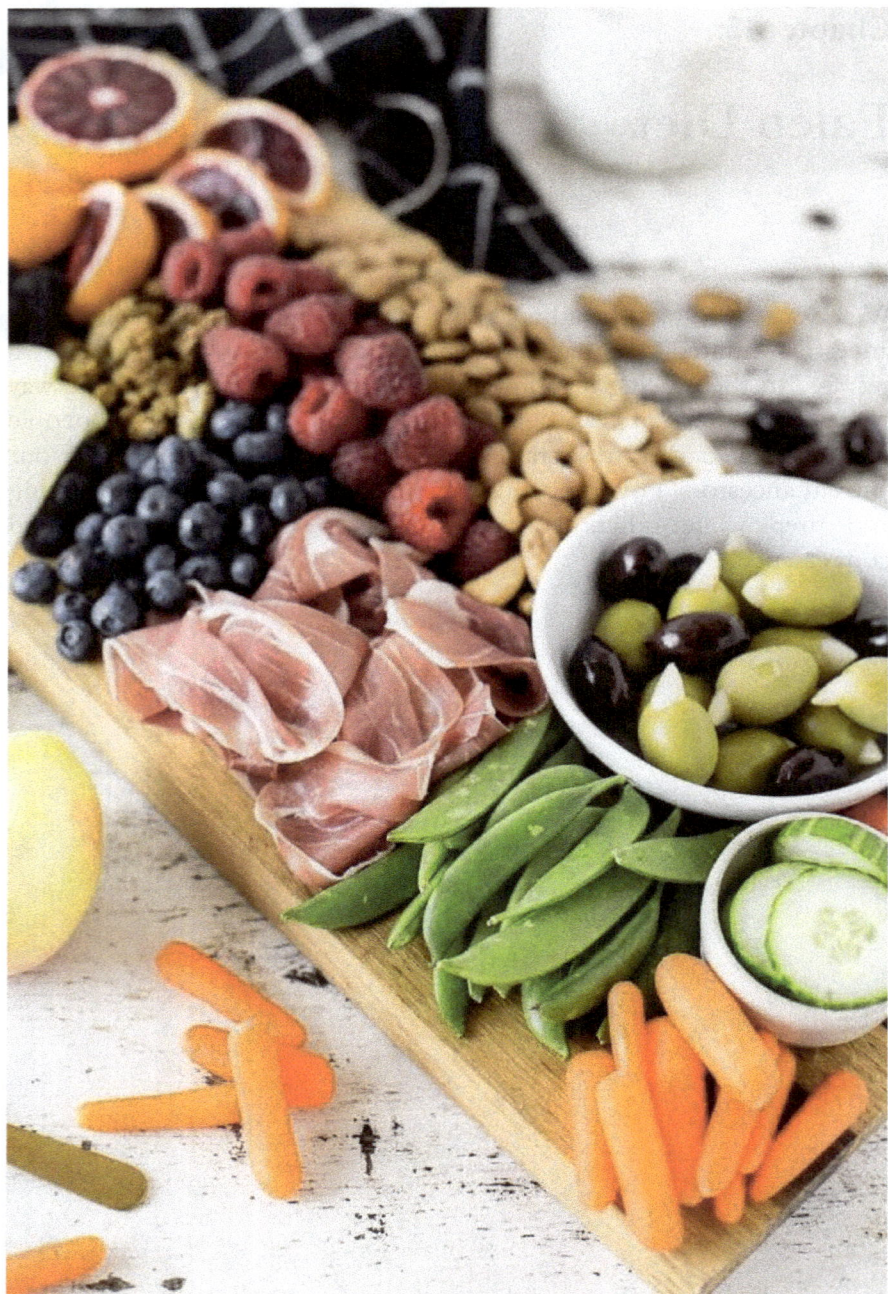

What Is the Paleo Diet?

The Paleo diet was created to mimic the way our ancestors ate based on the assumption that these are the foods our bodies were designed to ingest. The foods included in the diet are determined by what our ancestors hunted or gathered millions of years ago. A Paleo diet primarily consists of eating:

- meat (grass-fed or wild game)
- fish
- eggs
- vegetables
- nuts
- seeds
- fruits

Foods often avoided on the paleo diet include:

- dairy
- refined sugar
- legumes, beans, peanuts, peas
- salt
- processed foods
- artificial ingredients
- grains (rice, wheat, oats)
- potatoes

Many people incorporate fasting in with their paleo diet as our ancestors would have gone a few days here and there without eating. If fasting for a full 24 hours is not appealing, consider skipping a meal as our ancestors would have done.

Benefits

A Paleo diet is not for everyone but learning about the key benefits of this diet may make you change your mind. While much research still needs to be conducted, many people who make the switch to a paleo diet experience a wide range of benefits.

Weight Loss

The Paleo diet cuts out processed foods, excess carbohydrates, and sugar. Multiple studies indicate that when these items are removed and limited from one's diet there will be weight loss. Many studies have shown that individuals on a paleo diet see significantly more weight loss than with most other diets. Individuals may also reduce their waistline by more inches and decrease the amount of visceral body fat. Visceral body fat can lead to serious health problems as this fat wraps around the organs like the liver and intestines. The fat puts pressure on these organs and can overwork the system in the body. Decreasing this type of fat is essential for optimal health and will decrease one's risk for heart disease, obesity, and cardiovascular disease.

Cardiovascular Health

Many studies have been conducted that show how the Paleo diet can help improve cardiovascular health in a few key ways. It helps individuals raise HDL (good) cholesterol levels, lower triglyceride levels, decrease HbA1 levels, lose weight, reduce waist size, and lower blood pressure. One study compared the health benefits of the paleo diet against those of a standard diabetic diet. Individuals who followed a Paleo diet lost more weight, improved their HDL cholesterol levels, and lowered triglyceride levels. They also lost over six pounds more weight and decreased their waistline by four inches more than those who followed a standard diabetic diet (Jönsson et al., 2009).

Stabilize Blood Sugar Levels

The Paleo diet is low-carb so there is less need for insulin to constantly be pumped out from the pancreas. Those with type 2 diabetes or prediabetes can benefit from this diet because it helps improve insulin regulation and reduce the risk of insulin resistance.

Cons

Cutting out whole food groups like grains and dairy result in losing out on beneficial nutrients and fiber. In the long-term, removing these foods from one's diet can result in greater health risks.

The Paleo diet can be more complex to follow since it cuts out huge groups of standard foods most people consume daily. Additionally, while there are health benefits to this diet it does not outperform other diets that may be easier to follow.

The first month of the paleo diet is the hardest. During this month you are removing sugars, most carbs, and grain-based foods. This month can be riddled with ups and downs such as mood swings and low energy. It can be incredibly hard to stay motivated and stick with this eating plan in the beginning.

Eating out will also take more planning. It can be hard to find a place to dine out when you are on the paleo diet because so many menu items will include grains, dairy, and sugars. You will have to plan ahead to know what to order off the menu.

There can also be a negative impact on gut health. While the paleo diet can improve gut health in the short term, long-term adherence to the diet can cause an imbalance of the 'microbiome,' or gut bacteria. The paleo diet eliminates foods that can cause gut issues for those who have food allergies or food intolerances. Processed foods, gluten, wheat, and dairy are some of the most common culprits of digestive issues. These foods are known to increase inflammation in the digestive tract and body. Those on a paleo diet benefit from removing these foods, but the effects are only beneficial when sticking to the diet for less than a year. Those who continue with a paleo diet for more than a year can experience negative effects on gut health. Certain foods like legumes and whole grains promote diversification in the gut microbiome. When these foods are eliminated from one's diet for long periods of time, diversification of the gut microbiome decreases and pathogenic bacteria increase. This bacteria and others increase the risk of cardiovascular disease because it narrows the arteries in the body.

Getting Started

Always do your shopping with a grocery list. Having a list ensures you are sticking to paleo-approved foods. This shopping list will be your biggest tool for resisting temptation and staying on track while shopping.

When you go shopping, load up on vegetables. If it is within your budget choose organic foods. Organic foods will not be treated with harmful chemicals and often have better nutrient quality because there are stricter guidelines for soil quality and harvesting.

Prepare snacks and meals when you can. Planning meals—especially snacks—will eliminate mindless eating and help you stick with your diet plan. Make use of leftovers as lunches, snacks, or dinner for another day of the week

Do not overcomplicate it. The paleo diet is meant to be a simplified approach to eating better. Remember, our ancestors did not have all the conveniences we have today. With this reminder, you can look at choosing the right foods with a minimalist approach. Stick with simple flavors that you enjoy. You do not need to add many spices, herbs, or have a large variety of foods on your plate.

There is a good amount of leniency when following this diet plan. It can be incredibly hard to adhere to for the first month. When you make an adamant effort to continue with it you will see improvements in many areas of your life.

Be open to experimenting with new foods and cooking methods. A crockpot can become your best friend on this diet and makes sticking to the plan easier and more convenient. As you experiment, make a list of your go-to paleo recipes that you can rotate regularly in your meal planning.

Consider a detox or cleansing diet before going paleo. Ridding the body of built-up toxins can give you a fresh start on the paleo diet. Many people find that going through a cleanse gives them the motivation and discipline to start and stick with the paleo diet.

Finally, drink plenty of water. Water will help you digest your foods, ward off hunger, and eliminate unnecessary calories.

7-Day Meal Plan

Monday

Breakfast: Two scrambled eggs with bacon and a banana.

Lunch: Grilled chicken over mixed greens topped with vinaigrette.

Dinner: Beef kabobs (made with pineapple, bell pepper, onions, and mushrooms).

Tuesday

Breakfast: Spinach and mushroom omelet.

Lunch: Vegetable soup.

Dinner: Chicken stir-fry with cauliflower rice.

Wednesday

Breakfast: Fruit salad and nuts.

Lunch: Tuna and avocado over mixed greens with olive oil and vinegar.

Dinner: Meatballs and zucchini noodles.

Thursday

Breakfast: Butternut squash hash with ham.

Lunch: Two hard-boiled eggs and roasted vegetables.

Dinner: Pork chili (no beans).

Friday

Breakfast: Breakfast stuffed peppers.

Lunch: Fresh berries and nuts drizzled with coconut milk and maple syrup or honey.

Dinner: Herb crusted salmon with roasted beets and sweet potatoes.

Saturday

Breakfast: Tomato and basil frittata.

Lunch: Cajun chicken, roasted bell peppers and onions wrapped in a lettuce leaf.

Dinner: Stuffed cabbage.

Sunday

Breakfast: Sautéed vegetables (onions, mushroom, and spinach cooked in olive oil) with bacon or ham.

Lunch: Grilled chicken with steamed vegetables.

Dinner: Spaghetti squash with bacon, spinach, and red bell peppers topped with tomato sauce.

*Snacks can be eaten anytime between meals but should be limited to fresh berries and vegetables.

Chapter 14:

Raw Food Diet

The Raw Food diet is a straightforward diet that can make it easier to learn what to eat to lose weight. When you are limited to eating raw foods you eliminate a lot of the struggles those starting a diet face such as what to eat, how many calories something contains, and if it's healthy. The Raw Foods diet provides optimal nutrients so you not only will lose weight but will improve overall health. However, like any diet there are setbacks that you need to consider.

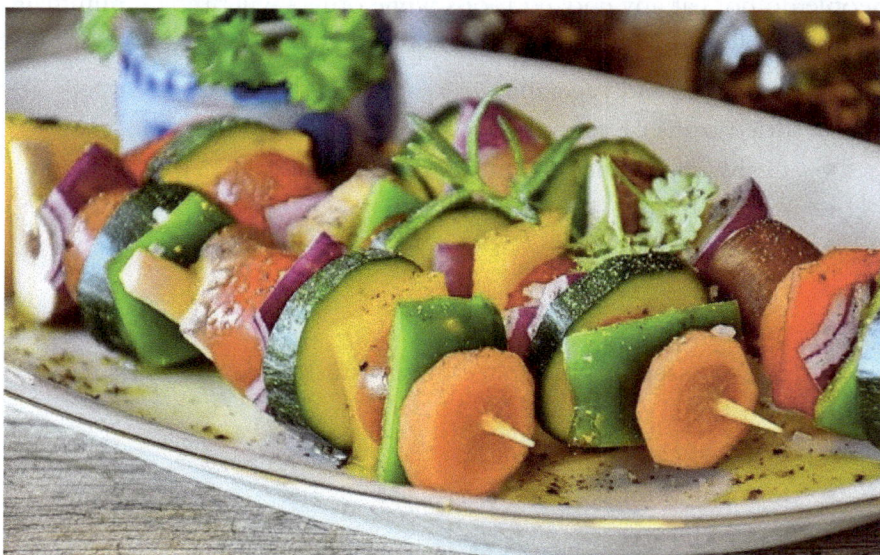

What Is the Raw Food Diet?

The Raw diet, as its name implies, focuses on a diet of raw foods with little to no cooking. This approach—keeping foods in their raw form—

is done to maintain the natural nutritional value of what you are consuming. Many foods lose nutrients when they are heated or cooked. Creating a diet plan that focuses on raw foods ensures you get all the benefits from what you eat.

There are three types of the Raw Food diet:

1. Raw Vegan diet: Includes plant-based foods and cuts out all animal products.
2. Raw Vegetarian diet: Includes all plant-based foods but allows raw eggs and any unprocessed dairy.
3. Raw Omnivorous diet: Includes plant-based foods, raw animal products, and allows raw or dried meat.

Each of these diets have flexibility in how foods are prepared. Some people do not eat any cooked foods while others will prepare minimally cooked meals. Foods that are allowed on the raw food diet include:

- raw fruits and vegetables
- dried fruits or vegetables
- freshly made juices (fruits or vegetables)
- soaked beans, legumes, and grains
- raw seeds and nuts
- raw nut butters
- nut milks
- cold pressed oils (like olive or coconut)
- nutritional yeast
- dried wheatgrass and algae
- fermented foods
- purified water
- unprocessed, organic, and natural foods
- sun-cured olives

If you are following a raw food diet and want to include some animal products you can incorporate the following:

- raw eggs
- raw fish

- raw meats
- dried meats
- non pasteurized, non homogenized milk and other dairy products.

Foods that are excluded from this diet include:
- cooked and processed foods
- refined oils
- refined sugars
- refined flour
- coffee
- tea
- alcohol
- table salt
- pasta
- canned or tinned olives
- tap water

Foods on the raw diet can be cooked but most adhere to preparing foods that have been cooked below 115°F. Other ways you can prepare foods on this diet include:
- soaking in water
- drying or dehydrating
- juicing or smoothies

Benefits

The Raw Food diet provides plenty of nutrients because it is high in fruits, vegetables, and nuts. You get even more nutrients because you are consuming these items raw so they maintain most of their nutritional value. These additional nutrients translate to additional health benefits.

Reduces Inflammation

When you transition to a raw food diet you will help cleanse the body of toxins and heavy metals which cause inflammation in the body. When you stick with eating primarily raw foods you will consume more enzymes that can help repair tissues in the body damaged by inflammation. The Raw Foods diet eliminates most foods that disrupt gut health and are not processed in the digestive tract properly which results in inflammation throughout the body. Many health care professionals recommend consuming more raw foods like fruits and vegetables to help those with chronic inflammatory conditions.

Decrease the Risk of Cardiovascular Disease

The raw food diet promotes healthy eating that helps lower blood pressure and increases good cholesterol levels. It is also a low-sodium diet that can reduce the risk of heart failure, kidney disease, type 2 diabetes, stroke, and other serious health issues.

Weight Loss

A raw food diet will help you lose weight for a number of reasons. You cut out the processed foods that can cause weight gain and you consume plenty of fruits and vegetables which are low in calories. Since this diet is rich in high-fiber foods, you will feel full longer so you will naturally eat less. When you combine all these factors you can expect to see weight loss.

Feel More Energized

When you fuel your body with clean, nutrient-rich foods, you will feel the difference. The Raw Food diet helps you feel less weighed down after eating. It provides a balance of essential macronutrients, vitamins, and minerals; this leads to feeling light and full of energy.

See Improvements With Your Skin

Getting rid of processed foods and consuming more nutritious foods will help heal your cells from the inside out. The Raw Food diet also encourages drinking plenty of water which is known to help skin look flawless.

Helps With Digestive Issues

Increasing the amount of fruit you eat—as recommended on the paleo diet—helps improve digestive function. Whole fruits contain plenty of fiber and other essential vitamins. The fiber helps slow down and support digestion while controlling appetite. Although the fiber slows down digestion it does not cause the foods you consume to sit in the digestive tract. Eating a plant-based diet leads to foods being processed and used more efficiently by the body.

Cons

There are some serious risks with the Raw Foods diet, especially when it comes to eating raw animal products. Consuming raw or undercooked meats, eggs, and fish, and raw or unpasteurized milk and dairy can result in food poisoning. Additional foods to prepare with caution include:

- Buckwheat; when consumed in large quantities can be toxic.
- Kidney beans and most legumes have phytic acid which blocks the body's ability to absorb certain minerals. Cooking the beans reduces the phytic acids, when left uncooked this chemical can be toxic.
- Sprouted seeds like alfalfa and bean sprouts can cause food poisoning. These foods harbor bacteria like Salmonella, E.coli, and Listeria.

- Yucca and gaplek—also referred to as cassava—should not be consumed raw as they are toxic. Only cooking these items thoroughly makes them safe to eat.
- Raw and undercooked eggs can contain Salmonella.
- Raw milk and dairy that are unpasteurized can contain Listeria.

It is important to educate yourself on the risk of eating certain foods raw.

While overcooking foods can decrease their nutritional value, cooking foods can also release certain nutrients like beta carotene and lycopene. The cooking process also kills off harmful bacteria like Salmonella.

Those who are not used to eating raw foods may suffer from digestive issues like cramping or gas. This is due to the increase in fiber consumption. Once your body gets used to taking in more fiber, these symptoms will often reduce or disappear.

Sticking with a raw food diet long-term can put you at greater risk for cardiovascular issues. Those who follow the diet for years tend to have higher levels of homocysteine (tHcy) which is influenced by vitamin B-12. The main sources of vitamin B-12 include dairy, poultry, fish, and red meat. Higher tHcy has been found in those who suffer from cardiovascular issues.

You will need to plan your meals more carefully to ensure you are getting the appropriate calories and nutrients that you need.

Getting Started

You do not have to eat everything raw. When you get started on a raw food diet, begin by increasing the number of raw foods you eat but still keep some cooked items on your menu. Aim for at least 75% of the food you consume to be raw while the other 25% can be cooked.

Stock up on nuts and seeds. These foods will be great for on-the-go snacks and to keep in the office or car.

Don't be afraid to experiment with various raw food recipes. Many have the misconception that eating a raw food diet is going to be bland and boring. With the right spices, herbs, and homemade sauce, you can transform your dish into delicious meals.

Start stocking your kitchen with the right raw food tools. You will need a high-speed blender and food processor to help create smoothies and sauces. Additional kitchen tools to consider are a spiralizer, mandolin, sushi roll mats, dehydrator, and a smoker. These items can help make eating a raw food diet more fun and versatile.

Plan your meals. Planning your meals is essential so you do not waste your fresh fruits and vegetables. Before you go shopping, know exactly what you are using your food for and when.

Keep track of what you eat. Tracking what you eat is done more to know what you prefer raw and what raw foods make you feel satiated. On a raw food diet, you can easily get stuck in eating the same foods the same way. To give yourself more options it is best to track what you are eating and rate your meals based on how much you like the taste and how filling your meals were. You also want to take note of how long you were able to go between meals so you get a better idea of what foods you want to eat more of so you feel full throughout the day.

7-Day Meal Plan

Monday

Breakfast: Green Smoothie (blend together two cups of water with two cups of spinach, two cups of kale, a cup of blueberries, a cup of blackberries, and a frozen banana).

Lunch: Salad of leafy greens, tomatoes, celery, bell peppers, avocados, and sunflower seeds, drizzled with cold-pressed olive oil and fresh-squeezed orange juice.

Dinner: Spinach salad with cucumbers, tomatoes, onions, and orange segments. Top with walnuts.

Tuesday

Breakfast: Fresh juice (use two apples, a cup of spinach, and two carrots) and macadamia nuts.

Lunch: Zucchini salad with cucumber, tomato, and avocado, drizzled with fresh orange juice.

Dinner: Gazpacho (blend together; 2 avocados, ½ cucumber, ½ cup fresh lime juice, a teaspoon of coriander, a teaspoon of turmeric, a teaspoon of cumin and a cup of water).

Wednesday

Breakfast: A cup of strawberries with coconut cream (you can make your own coconut cream by blending young coconut flesh).

Lunch: Banana Smoothie (blend together two bananas, a tablespoon of raw almond butter, a tablespoon of raw cocoa butter and ice).

Dinner: Dehydrated zucchini sticks with mixed greens and fresh fruit.

Thursday

Breakfast: Assorted berries and an avocado.

Lunch: Leafy greens with apple slices, orange slices, tomatoes, and sunflower seeds. Drizzle with vinegar and fresh citrus juice.

Dinner: Vegan pad thai.

Friday

Breakfast: Apple cinnamon chia seed pudding.

Lunch: Zucchini noodle salad with peanuts.

Dinner: Smoked salmon, cucumber, alfalfa sprouts, avocado, and red bell peppers wrapped in collard green leaves.

Saturday

Breakfast: Banana ice cream and fresh fruit.

Lunch: Dehydrated broccoli chips, raw cauliflower rice, and sliced mangos.

Dinner: Raw vegan tacos.

Sunday

Breakfast: Chocolate and raspberry chia seed pudding.

Lunch: Shredded brussel sprout salad.

Dinner: Zucchini noodles and spinach with a raw cashew alfredo sauce.

Chapter 15:

South Beach Diet

The South Beach diet was initially created to help lower the risk of heart disease. Though the diet came about in the 1990s, it became a popular diet for weight loss in the early 2000s. While the diet may not be talked about as much now as it used to be, many people recognize its name. The South beach diet can help you lose weight because it focuses on eating the right carbs, using a unique approach. The South Beach diet is a different approach to traditional low-carb diets and may assist you in your weight loss goals.

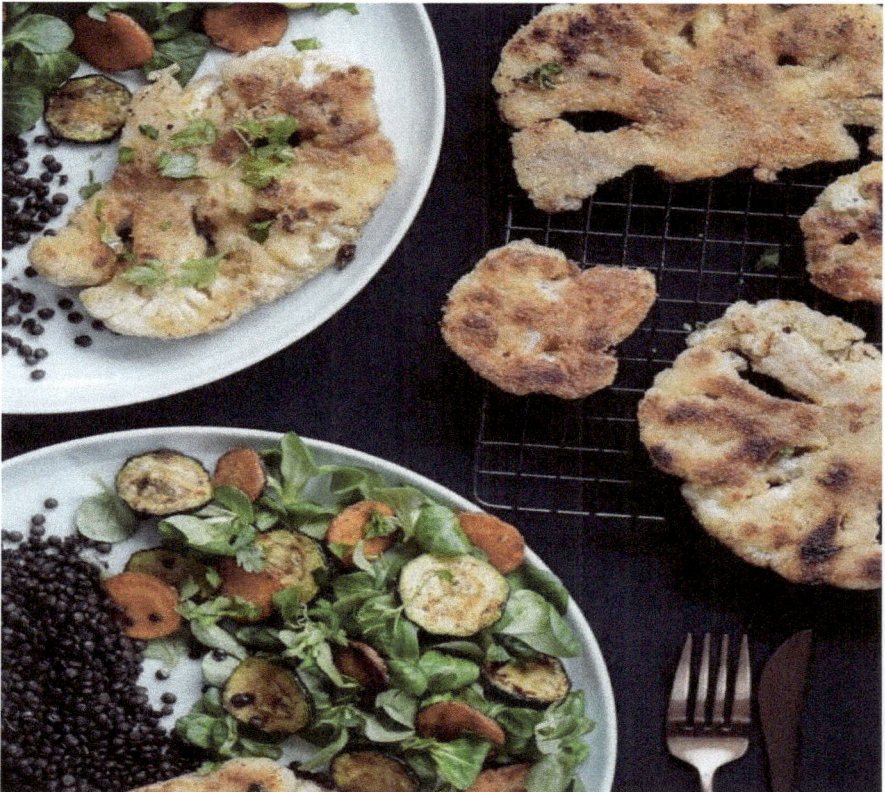

What Is the South Beach Diet?

While many have the assumption that the South Beach diet is another type of low-carb diet, it is not. The diet plan focuses on choosing the right types of carbs to include in your diet such as whole grains, some fruits, and vegetables. Other carbs are encouraged to be limited or avoided based on the glycemic index (GI) score.

The glycemic index lists foods based on how they increase blood sugar levels. Foods are classified as low, medium or high. Foods low on the index have a number value of 55 or less, medium index values will range from 56 to 60, foods considered high have a value of 70 or more. Many foods that fall in the high category have refined carbohydrates. These refined carbs are digested and absorbed through the body quickly causing blood sugar levels to spike.

There are three phases of the South Beach diet.

Phase one: This lasts for two weeks and is meant to kickstart weight loss. During this phase you will eliminate a few items from your diet, including:

- bread
- rice
- pasta
- potatoes
- pastries
- sugary foods
- fruit
- alcohol

The first phase is designed to help minimize cravings. You will eat three balanced meals a day and snacks. It is recommended that even if you are not necessarily hungry to still eat healthy snacks in between meals. Snacks are to keep you satisfied throughout the day and reduce the risk of overeating at meal times. Meals will consist of the following foods:

- lean meats
- poultry
- fish and shellfish
- tofu
- eggs
- nuts
- beans
- vegetables
- reduced fat cheese

Phase two: This will last until you have reached your desired healthy weight. In the first phase, you may experience rapid weight loss; in phase two you will still continue to lose weight but at a slow and steady pace. Steady weight loss in this phase is more likely to result in the weight remaining off.

During the second phase you will reintroduce good carbohydrates. The reintroduction of carbs will begin with just one new carb a week and only for one daily meal that week. For example, you can add fruit to your breakfast, but you will not eat fruit at another time during the day. When a carb is reintroduced you should monitor your body's response to the carb. Consider the following:

1. Do you feel more energized?
2. Do you have better quality sleep?
3. Is your mood better, or do you experience fewer irregular mood swings?
4. Are you still experiencing weight loss?
5. Is your digestion regular? Are you feeling less bloating, discomfort, or irregular bowel movements?
6. Is your skin more clear and healthy looking?

You want to closely monitor the reaction you have to these carbs. A negative reaction often indicates a spike in glucose levels and those foods you want to avoid. If you do not have a negative reaction to the carb, continue to add in another for a week. Continue this process until you have added two to three servings of carbs a day with no negative reactions. Remember, you should still be losing weight and you should not be having cravings while going through this process.

It is not uncommon for people to go back to phase one after they have reintroduced a few carbs. Consider returning to phase one if you experience:

- cravings
- trouble controlling portion sizes
- weight gain
- notice unhealthy eating habits re-emerge

You do not need to repeat phase one for another two weeks. Going back for a few days can help you regain control and plan out a new approach to phase two. Once you have reintroduced the recommended amount of healthy carbs to your diet and reached your goal weight, you can move on to phase three.

Phase three: This is a long-term phase. This phase is about maintaining your new habits and weight. During this final phase you are transitioning to a lifestyle of healthy eating habits. Take what you discovered from the second phase; learn which foods you can enjoy regularly and which you want to limit yourself to. Do not go back to eating as you used to before you began, instead, continue to make better food choices that result in better health and feeling better about yourself.

Benefits

The South Beach diet is a long-term approach to losing weight and keeping it off. The various phases provide different benefits and if the third phase is properly maintained, you can see significant improvements to your health. Read more about these benefits below.

Rapid Weight Loss in the First Phase

The South Beach diet claims that it can help you shed anywhere from 8 to 13 pounds in the first two weeks (Lee, 2021). During the second phase many people continue to lose one or two pounds a week as they begin to add foods back into their diet but still keep their calorie intake low.

Control Blood Sugar Levels

As a low-carb diet, it is expected that blood sugar levels will lower. The South Beach diet has shown to help regulate blood sugar levels and combat insulin resistance. The diet was originally created to help obese patients with heart disease improve their health and one of those key improvements focused on lower blood sugar levels. Individuals are encouraged to consume complex carbs on this diet—not completely eliminate them. Complex carbs do not cause blood sugar levels to spike, instead they provide a constant stream of energy to fuel the body with.

Maintain Target Weight for the Long-Term

The first phase helps promote rapid weight loss, but the other two phases assist with maintaining a healthy weight. Slowly adding healthy carbohydrates and fats into the diet allows individuals to learn how to eat so they are full and satisfied. This approach can help individuals manage their weight for the long-term. The diet also encourages incorporating exercise into your daily life. Adding physical activity to healthy diet changes not only results in more weight loss but ensures you keep the weight off.

Balanced Cholesterol Levels

The South Beach diet encourages eating foods low in saturated fats. When you begin to replace these saturated fats with heart-healthy unsaturated fats, cholesterol levels improve. Consuming nuts, seeds, and avocados in moderation increases HDL levels and will keep triglyceride levels low.

Reduce Cravings and Feel More Energized

During the first phase of the diet you will eliminate many foods that cause cravings like sugar and carbohydrates. You are replacing these with nutritious foods that will keep you feeling full. The reason your body has cravings for sugar or carbs is because it is lacking nutrients it needs to function and be fueled. When you are feeling low on energy many people crave carbohydrates (pasta and bread) when their body is really saying it needs protein. By supplying the body with what it needs, the cravings disappear and your risk for overeating and binging also reduces.

Cons

The first thing to point out is the South Beach diet was a very popular fad. There have been many claims about how effective it is when it comes to weight loss that may have been false. The reason it became popular so quickly was because of promises of rapid weight loss in just two weeks and other claims about certain foods causing weight gain. While there is some evidence that this diet can be effective, there are many more false claims that produce unrealistic expectations when on the diet.

Understanding the GI index is crucial for knowing which carbs to add during the second phase and which ones to avoid. While this index is fairly straight-forward you also have to take into consideration the serving size of that food item. Many people cut out certain carbs because they have a high GI but do not take note that it refers to a serving size you will most likely not consume in one sitting.

The second phase can be frustrating and requires patience while incorporating mindfulness into your day. You need to be more aware of how the carbs you reintroduce can have an impact on various activities during your day. Keeping track of the side effects can be just as cumbersome as counting calories. Though you will benefit greatly from understanding how your body responds to the foods you eat, this is not something most want to spend their time doing.

If you want to go with pre-packaged South Beach diet meals or meal plans, you might spend more than you expect. While these things can help you stick with the diet, many people rely on them instead of learning how to make their own meals. Not everyone has it in their budget to afford these meals or plans. For many, this may not be a budget friendly approach. If you rely on prepackaged meals, you may have to cut back your spending. This can lead to returning to unhealthy eating habits.

Getting Started

The first thing you want to do is understand the glycemic index. Get rid of foods in your home that are high on this list and shop for foods that are low on the index.

Come up with a system for tracking your weight loss and take measurements (sometimes the scale can be misleading and you may be losing inches but may not see the number of the scale moving).

Phase 1, 7-Day Meal Plan

Monday

Breakfast: Three egg whites with a cup of kale cooked in a tablespoon of olive oil.

Snack: An ounce of string cheese with a sliced bell pepper.

Lunch: Boneless sirloin burger topped with cheese and tomatoes; served with a side of three bean salad.

Snack: Celery sticks with two tablespoons of nut butter.

Dinner: Grilled steak and steamed broccoli.

Tuesday

Breakfast: Egg white, mushroom, and mozzarella cheese omelet with a side of Canadian bacon.

Snack: Pistachios and Swiss cheese.

Lunch: Mushroom soup.

Snack: Steamed broccoli and roasted chickpeas.

Dinner: Baked trout served with grilled asparagus and zucchini.

Wednesday

Breakfast: Green Smoothie (blend together ½ cup of almond milk, ½ cup of water, ½ an avocado, ½ cup of kale, ½ cup of spinach, and a tablespoon of almond butter).

Snack: Greek yogurt

Lunch: Tuna salad with cucumber and tomatoes.

Snack: Edamame and string cheese.

Dinner: Baked chicken breast stuffed with broccoli and cheese. Serve with a side of kale salad.

Thursday

Breakfast: Turkey on cloud bread.

Snack: A hard-boiled egg and tomatoes.

Lunch: Grilled chicken salad drizzled with balsamic vinaigrette.

Snack: Mixed nuts.

Dinner: Baked scallops with cauliflower mash and sautéed mushrooms.

Friday

Breakfast: Vegetable omelet.

Snack: Roasted chickpeas.

Lunch: Chicken avocado salad wrapped in lettuce.

Snack: Greek yogurt and cashews.

Dinner: Grilled salmon with grilled eggplant and mustard greens.

Saturday

Breakfast: Scrambled eggs, ham, and a side of cottage cheese.

Snack: Turkey and cheese roll ups.

Lunch: Grilled shrimp and spinach salad.

Snack: Mixed nuts.

Dinner: Garlic and ginger beef with broccoli.

Sunday

Breakfast: Hard boiled eggs, tomatoes, and avocado.

Snack: Zucchini boats with red bell pepper, tomatoes, and herbs.

Lunch: Chicken stir-fry with cauliflower rice.

Snack: Almonds and cheese.

Dinner: Salmon niçoise salad.

Phase 2, 7-Day Meal Plan

This meal plan incorporates adding just one new carb a day so it is ideal to use for your first week of the second phase. You can easily add in another serving of carbs each day such as a piece of fruit for a snack for the second week of phase two.

Monday

Breakfast: A cup of steel cut oats (made with water) with four tablespoons of peanut butter.

Snack: Cucumber slices with a quarter cup hummus.

Lunch: Grilled chicken salad.

Snack: Cottage cheese (add sliced peaches for the second week of phase two).

Dinner: Pork fajitas with a third cup of guacamole (use large lettuce leaves for the wrap).

Tuesday

Breakfast: Mushroom and cheese omelet.

Snack: Celery sticks with low-fat cream cheese.

Lunch: Tuna salad over mixed greens and tomatoes with a slice of whole-wheat bread.

Snack: Greek yogurt (add fresh berries for the second week).

Dinner: Roasted chicken with peppers and onions.

Wednesday

Breakfast: Whole-wheat toast with nut butter.

Snack: Hard-boiled egg and string cheese.

Lunch: Turkey, ham, and cheese rolled in a lettuce leaf.

Snack: Zucchini pizza bites.

Dinner: Burger bowl.

Thursday

Breakfast: Ham and cheddar egg muffins.

Snack: Greek yogurt with macadamia nuts.

Lunch: Cauliflower rice stuffed peppers.

Snack: Whole grain chips with salsa and guacamole.

Dinner: Zucchini Lasagna.

Friday

Breakfast: Scrambled eggs with zucchini tots.

Snack: Celery stick with cream cheese and sesame seeds.

Lunch: Stuffed sweet potato.

Snack: Cottage cheese with cucumber and salsa.

Dinner: Pan sheet chicken and vegetables served with kale salad.

Saturday

Breakfast: Oatmeal with cinnamon and walnuts (add apples after week one of phase two).

Snack: Ham and cheese roll ups.

Lunch: Shrimp scampi with zucchini noodles.

Snack: Nut and seeds mix.

Dinner: Beef and broccoli.

Sunday

Breakfast: Breakfast Smoothie (1 cup almond milk, ½ cup water, ¼ cup oats, ½ cup spinach, ½ an avocado and a tablespoon flaxseed). Add a cup of fresh berries after the first week of phase 2.

Snack: Mini bell peppers with cream cheese and chives.

Lunch: Shaved asparagus salad with almonds and balsamic reduction.

Snack: Kale chips and roasted chickpeas.

Dinner: Pan seared cod with roasted red peppers, black beans, and tomatoes.

Chapter 16:

Vegan

Veganism has gained in popularity over the years for many reasons. While focused around environmental factors and ridding the world of animal cruelty, a vegan diet has many health benefits. A vegan diet for most is not easy to transition to which is why most people adopt a strong 'why' for going vegan—such as to lower their carbon footprint, reduce the need for factory farmed animals, or preserve the Earth. If your reason for going vegan is just to lose weight, you may not have as much success or stick with the diet for long.

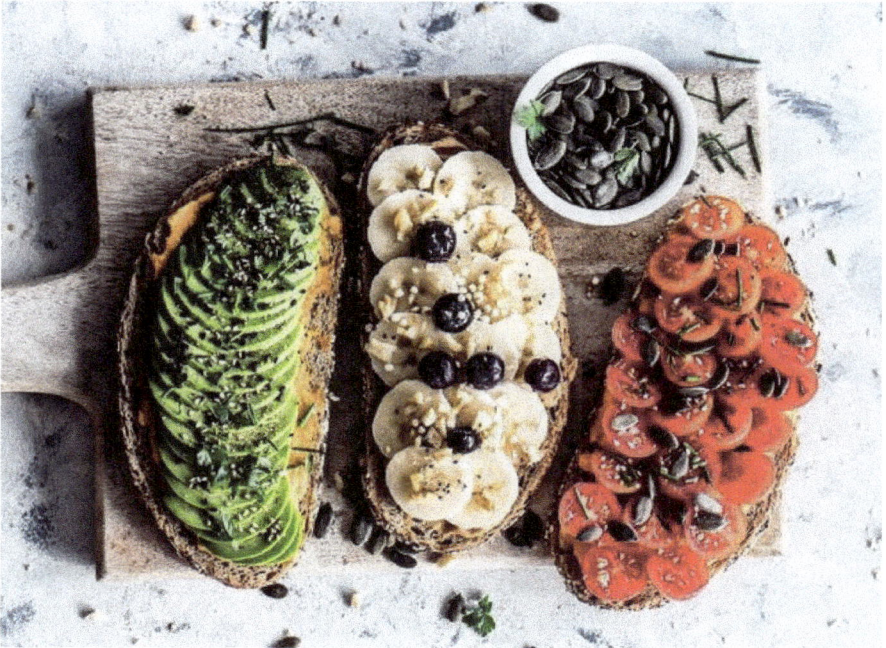

What Is the Vegan Diet?

Most who transition to a vegan diet do so for more than just health reasons. Vegans adopt this lifestyle because of the environmental impact. Veganism goes beyond cutting out animal products from your diet. Any items that are tested on animals, manufactured from animals (like leather and wool), or are obtained from the work of animals (like taking honey from bees) are eliminated.

On a vegan diet, you will not consume any animal products. This includes:

- meat, poultry, and seafood
- dairy
- eggs

There are plenty of vegan products you can use as an alternative to some of the previously mentioned non-vegan options. Foods you can consume on a vegan diet include:

- fruits
- vegetables
- tofu
- tempeh
- beans
- lentils
- nuts and nut butter
- seeds
- algae
- nutritional yeast
- whole grains
- sprouted and fermented plant food (Ezekiel bread, miso, kombucha)
- almond milk
- soy milk

There are many variations to a vegan diet and a lot of people find success with going vegan by combining it with another type of diet. For example, some vegans also combine a raw food diet with their meal planning where at least half their meals and foods will remain in raw form. You can choose how closely you follow a vegan lifestyle; while most vegans choose to eliminate all animal products or animal-tested products from their homes, others do not put as much emphasis on things outside of their diet.

Benefits

A vegan diet provides many health benefits but most of the scientific findings are inconclusive or contradictory. These results can be due to many factors as to how the studies done on a vegan diet are conducted (whether there was a control group or other lifestyle factors). While studies may not completely confirm the benefits of a vegan diet, that does not mean there are not many to experience. Below you will learn why a vegan diet might be an ideal choice for you.

Lose Weight

A vegan diet can help you lose more weight in the short term. Many studies have been conducted that show those who stuck with a vegan diet for six months lost more weight than those on a non-vegan diet (Turner-McGrievy et al., 2014). Weight loss is primarily due to an increase in eating more fresh fruits, vegetables, and whole grains while reducing the consumption of fat and saturated fats in addition to eliminating other non-vegan foods. Those starting out on a vegan diet can still expect to lose weight even if they do not follow the vegan diet perfectly. Making small adjustments to your diet and moving away from eating a Western diet can help you lose weight.

Plant-Based Benefits

A vegan diet provides you with the same health improvements as eating a plant-based diet. These can include:

- managing blood pressure
- decreased risk of type 2 diabetes

- reduced risk of hypertension
- protection against certain types of cancers.
- lowered cholesterol levels
- reduced risk of heart disease
- reduced risk of certain cancers

Cons

The main concern of going vegan is getting the essential vitamins and minerals your body needs. Many nutrients are easily available in plant-based products but some are consumed through non-plant based sources. These include:

- calcium
- vitamin B12
- vitamin D
- iron
- omega-3

A vegan diet does require more diligence. You need to be aware of everything you consume and ensure it falls into a vegan category. Going out to eat can be especially challenging and oftentimes impossible unless you dine out in a vegan establishment. If those you are going out to eat with are not also vegan, it can cause strain on some relationships and make you feel a little isolated because of your lifestyle choices.

Many vegan substitutes are not healthier than traditional items. Many companies are creating products that vegans can buy: meatless burgers, dairy made from soy, and other alternatives. While these give you options for enjoying some of the traditional foods you are used to, they are often highly processed and made from questionable ingredients. These vegan options do not provide additional health benefits. There are vegans who are overweight and this is primarily due to not properly planning their meals or paying attention to food labels.

A vegan diet may significantly restrict your food options. Remember that a vegan diet does not just eliminate animal food sources but also animal by-product ingredients. Nearly all meals contain at least one animal by-product, making it challenging to prepare meals for those not accustomed to this way of eating.

Getting Started

There are many things you may need to cut from your diet. You can go all in and cut everything all at once but many have more success cutting one group of foods at a time. Begin by cutting back on your meat intake. Start with one meatless day a week and stick with this for two to four weeks, then go meatless two days and so on. Once you've done that, begin to cut out another group such as dairy. Take the same approach and go dairy-free one day a week, then two, until you have cut it out of your diet completely. Remember, it is not just about eliminating these items but also finding sensible plant-based alternatives. For example, you can cut out dairy but still enjoy almond milk or oat milk. Additional things to keep in mind include:

- Experiment with different plant-based sources.
- Know how to make simple substitutions that are healthy.
- Always read the labels. Many products you buy in the store may contain animal by-products or non vegan ingredients like casein or whey protein isolate.

7-Day Meal Plan

If you feel hungry in between meals you can eat raw vegetables, a piece of fruit, or nuts and seeds.

Monday

Breakfast: Baked oatmeal with bananas and walnuts.

Lunch: Vegan chili.

Dinner: Soy-rizo tacos with mango pineapple salsa.

Tuesday

Breakfast: Tofu breakfast scramble.

Lunch: Vegetable sushi rolls and edamame.

Dinner: Loaded sweet potatoes and black beans.

Wednesday

Breakfast: Breakfast Smoothie (blend together a cup of almond milk. ½ cup of mangoes, a cup of spinach or kale).

Lunch: Lentil soup with kale.

Dinner: Tempeh stir-fry with broccoli and bok choy.

Thursday

Breakfast: Chickpea pancakes topped with fresh salsa and avocado.

Lunch: Tofu and green bean curry with cauliflower rice.

Dinner: Vegan shepherd's pie (made with mushrooms instead of ground beef).

Friday

Breakfast: Avocado, crispy tofu, and chickpeas wrapped in collard greens.

Lunch: Quinoa salad with chickpeas, tomatoes, and olives.

Dinner: Vegan Bombay burritos (roasted cauliflower and chickpeas with a potato and onion yellow curry spread).

Saturday

Breakfast: Banana pancakes topped with fresh berries and walnuts.

Lunch: Quinoa and black bean stuffed peppers.

Dinner: Tofu teriyaki with broccoli, cashews, and wild rice.

Sunday

Breakfast: Breakfast Smoothie (blend together a cup of soy milk, ½ cup of blueberries, 4 ounces of silken tofu, ½ cup of pineapples and a cup of spinach).

Lunch: White bean soup.

Dinner: Cauliflower steaks with pesto zucchini noodles.

Chapter 17:

Vegetarian Diet

Many people use vegan and vegetarian interchangeably, but the two diets have so many key differences. Vegan is a type of vegetarian diet but there are other options as well. Some vegetarians eat eggs, others won't. Some vegetarians will eat fish but stay away from red meat and poultry. A vegetarian diet can be flexible but there is a focus on eating primarily plant-based foods. Read on to learn more about how you can easily transition to a vegetarian diet and take better control of your diet and health.

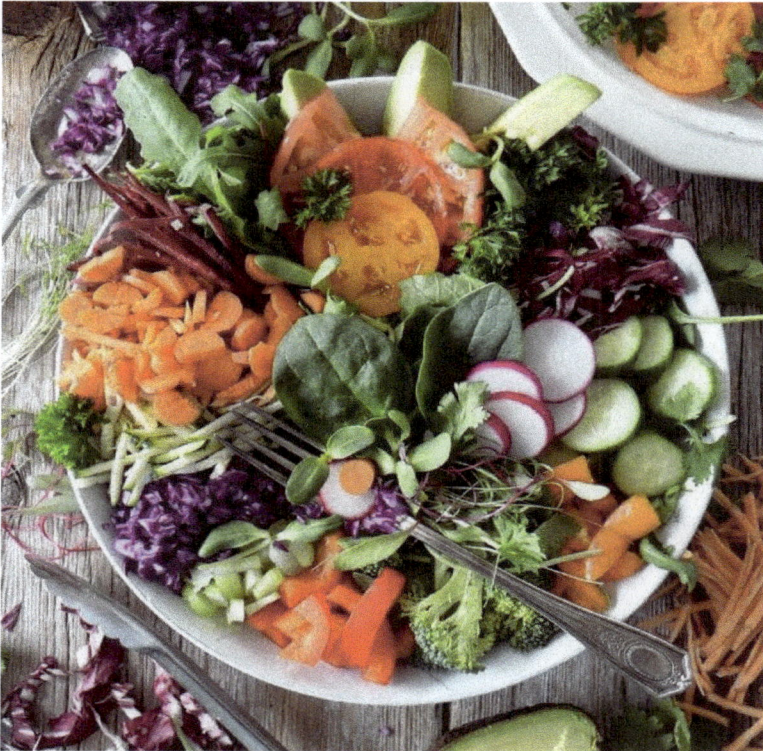

What Is a Vegetarian Diet?

Vegetarian diets focus on plant-based food sources, though there are many variations of vegetarian diets that may better suit your lifestyle. The vegan diet, flexitarian diet, and Mediterranean diet are some examples of vegetarian diets. There are five common types of vegetarian diets, which include:

- Lacto-vegetarian: excludes meat, fish, poultry, and eggs but does allow for dairy products.
- Ovo-vegetarian: excludes meat, poultry, fish, seafood, and dairy but does allow eggs.
- Lacto-ovo vegetarian: excludes meat, fish, and poultry, but does allow dairy and eggs.
- Pescatarian: excludes meat, poultry, dairy, and eggs but does allow fish.
- Vegan: excludes all animal products and by-products.

There is no one size fits all when it comes to vegetarian diets, though there is a common consensus that your diet is primarily made of:

- fruits
- vegetables
- low-fat dairy or plant-based alternative
- beans, lentils, legumes
- unsaturated oils (sunflower oil, vegetable oil, flaxseed oil)
- tofu
- tempeh

Foods chosen should be low in salt, fat, and sugar.

Benefits

Even if you do not commit to a fully vegetarian diet and instead opt to include eggs or dairy, you will still be taking vital steps to improve your health. A vegetarian diet has been shown to provide many positive results when it comes to weight loss and various chronic conditions. Below, you will learn about a few key benefits you can expect to experience when switching to a vegetarian diet.

Weight Loss and Weight Management

Since a vegetarian diet is primarily made up of vegetables and fruit, you are consuming more low-calorie foods. Fewer calories helps you lose weight and keep it off.

Reduce the Risk of Serious Health Conditions

Vegetarian diets are typically low in saturated fat and sugar. Both of these have been linked to an increased risk of cardiovascular disease, obesity, high blood pressure, and heart disease. Studies have shown that individuals who consume a plant-based diet had more than a 70% decrease in cardiovascular disease (Stein, 2018).

Reduce the Risk of Certain Cancers

Eliminating red meat from your diet reduces the number of carcinogens that can build up in the colon. Studies have shown that vegetarians are at less risk for developing colon cancer for this reason, among others.

Increase in Life Expectancy

A long-term study conducted at Loma Linda University showed that those who ate a vegetarian diet outlived their non-vegetarian counterparts (those who ate a primarily carnivorous diet). The study lasted over 14 years and tracked the lifestyle and diets of 34,000 participants, determining that women who consumed a vegetarian diet live six years longer than non-vegetarians. Men lived for nearly a decade longer. (Can Eating A Vegetarian Diet Really Help You Live Longer?, n.d.). Other research has backed this information showing a vegetarian diet provides individuals with essential fiber and highly beneficial plant compounds like antioxidants and phytochemicals. These factors, among others, help improve overall health which will add years to your lifespan.

Cons

You need to be aware of the vitamins and minerals you consume. As we have discussed with other vegetarian diets, there is concern over getting adequate nutrients. If you are cutting out animal products, you need to understand where to get the right balance of nutrients in your plant-based options.

Excluding certain food groups can put you at a greater risk of a decrease in muscle mass. Meat is essential for growing and maintaining muscle mass because the body needs the protein in meat to fuel those muscles. When you switch to a vegetarian diet and eliminate meat, you may struggle to maintain muscle mass.

Be careful about eating too many soy products. Many vegetarians use soy products as meat and dairy alternatives. Many soy-based products are created from genetically modified plants and these can be harmful.

You also cut out foods that supply you with calcium. Calcium is essential for bone health and most vegetarians do not get enough calcium through their diet. Unless you are sticking with a lacto-vegetarian diet and consuming some dairy, there is a good chance that you're not getting the calcium your body needs. This lack of calcium can be more problematic for women who are at greater risk of osteoporosis. Though many vegetables contain calcium, most also contain oxalates which makes it harder for the body to absorb calcium.

Getting Started

Getting started on a vegetarian diet does not have to mean eliminating all animal products at once. The best way to start a vegetarian diet is to tackle one day or meal at a time. Much like the flexitarian diet, you can start off with going vegetarian for just one day a week and then slowly increase from there.

It is also recommended that you transform your favorite recipes into vegetarian alternatives. Begin to leave out meat from your favorite recipes and replace them with plant-based sources. For example, you can still enjoy your favorite chili recipes but instead of meat add in black beans or increase the number of beans you already include. If you love tacos, use sautéed mushrooms instead of ground meat.

You can begin by adding more vegetables to every meal and eat them first. If you double your vegetables or fruit with your meals you can cut your meat products in half. Getting used to having more vegetables on your plate and focusing on them first will ensure you eat more of them.

Finally, try to learn a few simple substitutions in recipes. In the meal plan below you will see a few options that you would typically need eggs, cream, or other non-vegetarian ingredients to make. Some of your favorite recipes probably contain them and this doesn't mean you never get to eat these dishes again. Knowing how to swap out the ingredients you do not want to eat with vegetarian options will allow you to still enjoy the meals you love. Some of the most basic substitutions to try, include:

- Mix one tablespoon of ground flaxseed with three tablespoons of water. Let the mixture sit for five minutes. You can use this to replace eggs in desserts, pastries, and other recipes where egg is used as a binder.
- Mashed banana and applesauce are two more egg replacement options that work well in cakes, muffins, and cookie recipes.
- Almond milk, soy milk, oat milk, and rice milk can be used instead of traditional cow's milk. You can make your own oat milk by blending ½ cup whole oats with 3 cups of water. Blend for 30 seconds then strain. If you want slightly sweeter milk, you can add 1 teaspoon of pure maple syrup. For vanilla flavor,

add ½ teaspoon of pure vanilla extract. Store in the refrigerator for up to 7 days.

- Nutritional yeast can be used to replace Parmesan cheese or can be added to recipes you want to add a cheese flavor to.
- Coconut cream can be used in place of regular cream. To make coconut cream, you just need to chill a can of coconut milk, the cream will form as a thick layer at the top of the can. Scoop this cream and use it in soups or in place of yogurt. You can also use an electric mixture to beat the cream into a coconut whipped cream.
- Mushrooms of any variety can be chopped and used in place of ground beef for tacos, burritos, and meaty pasta sauces.
- Jackfruit, which is found canned in most grocery stores, makes a great ground meat and shredded pork substitute.
- Reserve the water drained from your chickpea cans. Commonly called aquafaba, this liquid can substitute eggs in meringues, mousses, sponge cakes, and frosting recipes like royal icing.
- Cashews that have been soaked for at least four hours can be used to create cheese sauces.

7-Day Meal Plan

This is a traditional vegetarian meal plan, there are no eggs or dairy items used in any of the meals.

Monday

Breakfast: Oatmeal waffles topped with fresh fruit

Snack: Green Smoothie (blend together 1 cup of almond milk, 1 cup of kale, ½ cup of blueberries, and ½ cup of pineapples).

Lunch: Sweet potatoes, cranberry, and spinach salad. (add a hard-boiled egg if you want).

Snack: Mini sweet peppers filled with cream cheese and chives or hummus.

Dinner: Gnocchi with summer vegetables.

Snack: A Banana and nut butter.

Tuesday

Breakfast: Fruit and nut parfait (made with coconut cream).

Snack: An orange and walnuts.

Lunch: Sweet potato and chickpea pitas.

Snack: Tomato bruschetta.

Dinner: Stuffed portobello mushroom (filled with sautéed spinach, onions, and mushrooms) served with rice and beans.

Snack: Peach cobbler.

Wednesday

Breakfast: Blueberry pancakes.

Snack: Fruit bowl.

Lunch: Corn chowder (made with coconut cream).

Snack: Veggie sticks and hummus.

Dinner: Vegetarian enchiladas.

Snack: Baked apples and roasted pecans.

Thursday

Breakfast: Banana walnut muffin.

Snack: Rice cakes with nut butter.

Lunch: Quinoa-stuffed squash boats.

Snack: Tortilla chips and guacamole or salsa.

Dinner: Vegetarian pad thai.

Snack: Raspberry sorbet or sherbet.

Friday

Breakfast: Tofu scramble.

Snack: Roasted broad beans or Fava beans.

Lunch: Spinach and tomato quesadillas.

Snack: Avocado toast.

Dinner: Bean burger with sweet potato fries.

Snack: Fresh berries.

Saturday

Breakfast: Chocolate, blueberry, and almond oatmeal.

Snack: Celery and bell pepper sticks with guacamole.

Lunch: Kale and squash salad.

Snack: Fruit and nut trail mix.

Dinner: Vegetable stir-fry with brown rice noodles (add a cooked egg if desired).

Snack: Sliced apples and nut butter.

Sunday

Breakfast: Sprouted waffles with nut butter and banana.

Snack: Granola or oat bar.

Lunch: Lentil soup.

Snack: Falafel.

Dinner: Vegetarian lasagna.

Snack: Fruit Smoothie (blend together 1 cup of almond milk, ½ cup of mixed berries, ½ a banana, 1 teaspoon of maple syrup, and ¼ cup of rolled oats).

Chapter 18:

Volumetrics Diet

The volumetrics diet is a unique approach to eating healthy. It encourages you to choose foods that are filling and nutritious so you can lose weight and improve your health without having to make drastic changes all at once. You learn to eat more and feel satisfied without worrying about consuming excess calories that will add on the pounds. This eating approach eliminates the fear of having to deprive yourself of foods you love and instead, focuses on eating more of the foods that will make you feel good. No foods are off limits which is why many people find this diet to be highly beneficial in their weight loss journey.

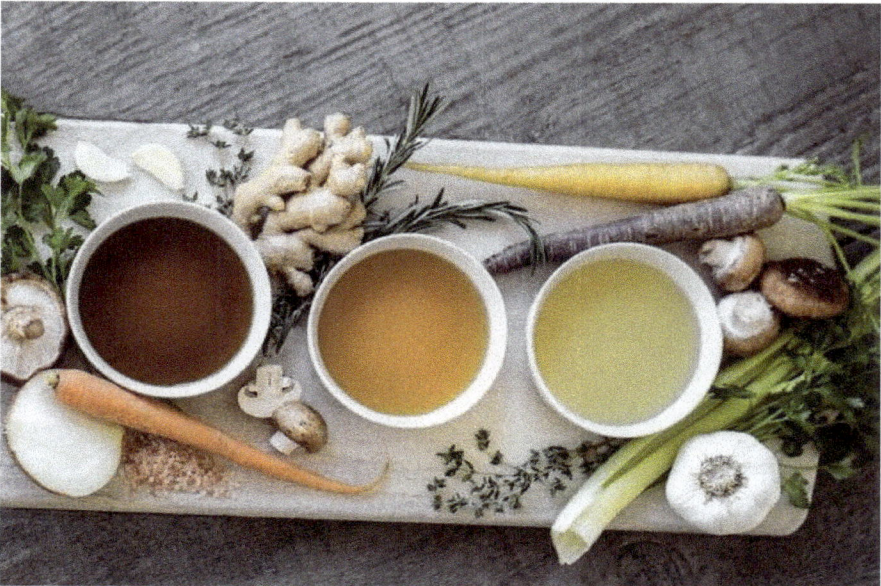

What Is the Volumetrics Diet?

The Volumetrics diet focuses on eating low-calorie foods that keep you feeling full. This approach to eating lets you fill up on higher quantities of food but without the risk of gaining weight. Other diets map out food to eliminate, foods to eat, and portion sizes, but they do not provide individuals with a solution when they feel hungry.

The volumetrics diet teaches you what foods will keep you feeling satiated for longer. Foods are categorized into four groups: very low energy dense foods, low energy dense foods, medium energy dense foods, and high energy dense foods. Very low energy-dense foods are considered to have a low density and calories but are high in nutrients. Fruit, non starchy vegetables, broth-based soups, and low-fat dairy would fall in the very low energy-dense foods category. These are considered very low-density and you can eat freely unless you are full. High energy dense foods are considered to have high calories and require you to eat a lot of them to feel full. These foods include butter, cookies, candy, and crackers. Most of the foods in this category are high in fat, sugar, and carbs. High density foods should only be consumed occasionally.

On the volumetrics diet, you will stick with foods in the very low density and low density groups. These foods include:

- fruit
- vegetables (choose non-starchy ones)
- low-fat dairy (Greek yogurt, kefir, cottage cheese)
- fiber-rich unprocessed whole grains (oats, brown rice, quinoa)
- lean protein (egg whites, tofu, extra-lean ground beef and pork, skinless chicken breast)

Foods that are avoided on the volumetrics diet include:

- full-fat dairy (full-fat yogurt, sour cream)
- fatty meat (bacon, sausages, regular ground beef)
- processed, refined, or sweetened foods (white bread, sugar cereal, candy, cakes, fried foods, sweetened drinks)

Benefits

The volumetric diet provides a much different approach to eating then the others diets mentioned so far. It also provides a whole solution to losing weight and maintaining optimal health. In this section you will learn how this different approach can provide you with more benefits.

Easy to Follow and Flexible

No foods are completely off limits. If you want to treat yourself to a piece of chocolate, you can, but you do need to stay within a calorie recommendation for the day. Those who struggle with highly restrictive diets that cut out food groups may benefit from this type of diet approach. The diet is also meant to be adopted as a life-long eating habit. Once you have reached your goal weight, you maintain it by increasing your portion size slightly or adding in an extra snack. You will still adhere to the same way of meal planning as you did when trying to lose weight.

Weight Loss

The volumetrics diet is highly effective for weight loss. The plan is designed to have you fill up on low-calorie but nutrient dense foods. This gives you better control over your appetite as you should feel full and more satisfied even though you are not consuming as many calories. When you cut back on calorie intake while still fueling your body with essential nutrients, you will lose weight in a healthy sustainable way.

Encourages Exercise

A balanced diet and exercise helps you burn off more fat and maintain a healthy lifestyle for the long-term. The volumetrics diet encourages individuals to get a minimum of 30 minutes of exercise daily and this can be any form of physical activity that you enjoy. Exercise is an important part of overall health and when added to a healthy diet you will be more energized and fit.

Helps Curb Appetite

A huge part of losing weight and keeping it off is eating so that you feel satiated throughout the day. Many high-calorie foods may fill you up quickly but won't keep you full for long, or you may need to eat a greater amount of these high-calorie foods to feel full. Eating these calorie dense foods will lead to weight gain because of the calorie intake and you never feel satiated. On the volumetrics diet you learn how to consume lower-calorie foods and you can eat as much of these as you want because the calorie intake remains low but they fill you. Studies have shown that individuals who followed a low calorie meal plan had fewer cravings, felt more full throughout the day, and reduced feelings of hunger (Buckland et al., 2018).

Cons

There is a lot of emphasis on how many calories are in the foods you eat. While effective, having to check the calorie content of everything you consume can be frustrating and overwhelming. You need to keep track of everything you eat via a food journal or calorie counting app to help track daily calories. This can be tedious and some personality types can become obsessed with tracking and counting their calories to the point that it begins to interfere with their daily lives.

The diet doesn't encourage the consumption of nuts and healthy fats like olive oil because of their higher calorie count. These items; however, have plenty of nutrients the body can benefit from. While these foods are not completely cut out, they are highly restricted and this may not be the best for overall optimal health.

It can be hard to dine out when adopting the volumetrics diet as most restaurants will cook with oil or butter. These items should be limited when on the volumetrics diet. You will need to plan ahead before dining out to ensure you can eat something on the menu. Sticking to a diet like this can become isolating as you may not find many places that fit in with your eating plan.

Getting Started

Get in tune with the cues your body gives you. When you are feeling hungry, it is okay to eat but stick with fruit and vegetables. When you are done eating a meal, give yourself 30 minutes before you go for seconds. It takes the body some time to cue the brain that it is full, which is why many people overeat in a short period of time and then are stuffed and uncomfortable from eating too much. Giving your body time to process the food you consume can help you eliminate unnecessary calories and help you feel better after you eat.

Try to plan your meals. You should be eating three meals a day and allow for one or two snacks in-between meals. Taking the time to create a menu for the week will help you know exactly what you're going to eat and when so that you remain full from one meal to the next.

Those looking to lose weight should weigh themselves once a week to track their progress. Weekly weigh-ins while keeping a food journal can help you identify foods that may cause you to keep weight on or add weight.

Incorporate a few days of exercise. To get the most out of the volumetrics diet for weight loss you need to add exercise into your routine. Aim to walk for 10 minutes, do 10 to 20 sit-ups, or track your steps. A little increase in your physical activity can lead to greater weight loss.

Additional tips to consider:

- Add more salads and broth-based soups to your daily meals. However, be careful about the toppings you add, like dressing which can increase the calorie content.
- You do not have to cut out your favorite foods. You can still enjoy your pasta but you want to swap out half the pasta for vegetables like broccoli and spinach.
- Avoid drinking your calories; instead of high sugar drinks stick with water, tea, or seltzer.
- Add nutrient-rich fruits to dense foods like cereal, low-fat yogurt, and oats.
- Keep a food journal that will help you learn which foods keep you full longer.
- Choose foods that are high in fiber. Fiber naturally makes you feel full and will keep you feeling full for longer periods of time.
- Stick with foods that have high water concentrations like broccoli, bell peppers, and melons.

7-Day Meal Plan

Monday

Breakfast: Vegetable omelet with a slice of whole-wheat toast.

Snack: Low-fat Greek yogurt and fresh fruit.

Lunch: Chili with vegetables, lean meat, and beans.

Snack: Air-popped popcorn (no butter or salt).

Dinner: Baked fish, steamed carrots, broccoli, and cauliflower. Served with quinoa.

Tuesday

Breakfast: Baked blueberry oatmeal.

Snack: A Banana, nut butter, and rice cakes.

Lunch: Vegetable soup with beans.

Snack: Vegetable sticks and hummus.

Dinner: Grilled chicken, roasted small potatoes, and cabbage.

Wednesday

Breakfast: Oatmeal with a banana and a few walnuts.

Snack: Low-fat cottage cheese and sliced fruit.

Lunch: Minestrone soup and a whole-grain roll.

Snack: Rice cakes and pineapple.

Dinner: Baked cod with steamed vegetables and couscous.

Thursday

Breakfast: Mushroom and spinach omelet with a slice of whole-wheat toast.

Snack: Fruit parfait.

Lunch: Lentil soup.

Snack: Pistachios and fresh berries.

Dinner: Roasted vegetables (zucchini, mushrooms, broccoli, and onions) with whole grain pasta and turkey meatballs.

Friday

Breakfast: Oatmeal with apples and cinnamon.

Snack: A hard boiled egg and banana.

Lunch: Grilled vegetable salad (eggplant, zucchini, bell pepper, and onions) with vinaigrette dressing.

Snack: Apple slices and low-fat cheese.

Dinner: Black bean or turkey burger with grilled zucchini sticks.

Saturday

Breakfast: Scrambled eggs with sautéed spinach, bell pepper, mushroom, and onions. Serve with a side of cantaloupe.

Snack: Blueberries and low-fat Greek yogurt.

Lunch: Grilled shrimp salad with tomatoes, cucumber, celery, and radish. Top with a vinaigrette dressing.

Snack: Bruschetta with tomatoes, onions, and peppers.

Dinner: Stuffed bell peppers with beans and quinoa.

Sunday

Breakfast: Whole-wheat pancakes with fresh berries.

Snack: Green Smoothie (blend together 1 cup of almond milk, ½ cup of kale, ½ cup of spinach, half an avocado, strawberries, pineapples, and blueberries).

Lunch: Tuna salad with spinach, tomatoes, cucumber, celery, and onions with a whole wheat pita and a side of cantaloupe.

Snack: Puffed rice cereal with low-fat milk topped with bananas or strawberries.

Dinner: Baked salmon with cauliflower mash, steamed broccoli, snow peas, and carrots.

Chapter 19:

Whole-Foods Plant-Based Diet

A whole-foods plant-based diet focuses on one key principle: to eat more natural foods. Those who may have struggled with losing weight or sticking to a diet plan may find a whole-foods plant-based approach to eating beneficial. The diet eliminates foods known to add on pounds and increase the risk of poor health. Aside from emphasizing eating real food over processed foods, it encourages you to eat delicious foods. This is done by adding spices, herbs, and creating your own sauces for your meal instead of relying on store-bought or pre-packaged items. Many people love the whole-foods plant-based diet because it is straightforward and easy to apply to daily life. Read on to learn how this diet approach can become a healthy lifestyle choice for you.

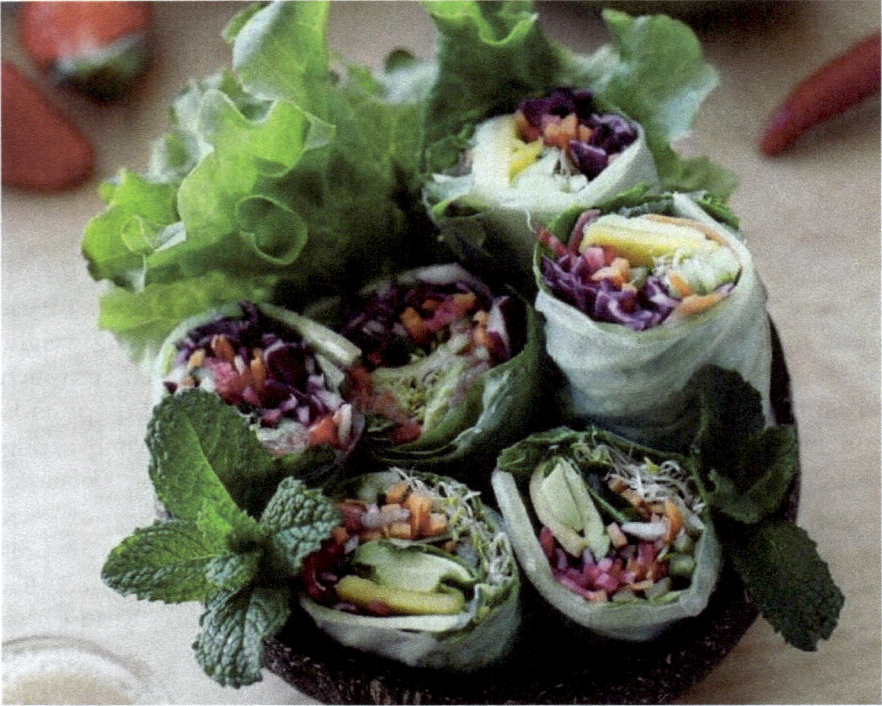

What Is the Whole-Foods Plant-Based Diet?

A whole-foods plant-based diet encourages you to freely eat fruits, vegetables, and legumes until you are full. Foods should be minimally processed. Many who transition to a whole-foods plant-based diet quickly adopt this as a lifestyle choice. They begin to bring more awareness to how food makes them feel and decide to incorporate more of the foods that keep them energized and feeling good.

A whole-foods plant-based diet follows a simple rule: eat more whole, unrefined, and plant-based foods. Food you can eat when you want and until you are full include:

- All vegetables, including root vegetables (fresh or frozen)
- legumes (dried or canned)

- whole grains (millet, quinoa, steel cut or rolled oats, brown rice, barley)
- fruit (fresh or frozen)
- omega 3 rich seeds (chia and flaxseed)
- spices
- unsweetened plant-based milks
- herbal teas
- decaffeinated coffee
- water

It is suggested that some foods be eaten occasionally. These include:
- nuts (almonds, cashews, walnuts, and nut butters)
- coconut (raw, unsweetened shredded coconut flakes, low-fat coconut milk)
- seeds (pumpkin, sunflower, sesame)
- dried fruits
- sweeteners (maple syrup, molasses)
- minimally processed soy products (tofu, miso, tempeh)
- caffeinated coffee
- alcohol

Foods that are avoided on a plant-based whole-foods diet include:
- meat including processed meats
- poultry
- seafood
- dairy
- eggs
- plant fragment or vegan replacement foods
- added fats (oil and margarine)
- refined sugar (white table sugar, corn syrup, cane sugar, beet sugar, brown rice sugar)
- refined grains (white flour, white rice, instant oats)
- protein isolates (soy protein and pea protein isolates, seitan)
- soda

- fruit juices
- energy drinks
- sports drinks

The idea is not to get caught up on the things you want to avoid or eliminate from your diet. Instead, you should focus on being able to eat more filling, satisfying, and nutritious foods. Keep in mind that many people on a whole-foods plant-based diet do incorporate meat, poultry, and fish into their diet. However, red meats need to be from organic grass-fed animals, poultry should be organic and free range, and fish should be wild caught.

Benefits

A whole-foods plant-based diet eliminates all the low-quality foods we consume that cause us to gain weight and see a decline in our health. While a whole-foods plant-based diet is similar to a vegetarian diet, flexitarian diet, and even vegan diet, each of these diets allow for more flexibility to consume processed items. Since the whole-foods plant-based diet encourages making more of your own foods to completely eliminate the need for store bought packaged items, you will see more benefits with this diet approach.

Reduce the Risk of Cancers

A whole-foods plant-based diet lowers the risk of certain cancers like prostate and breast cancer. Cutting out preservatives, added sugar, and other modified foods from your diet will eliminate free-radicals and excess toxins in your system. These items can increase your chance of developing certain types of cancers.

Prevent and Help Treat Heart Disease

Consuming more whole foods packed with antioxidants, nutrients, and minerals is a cornerstone for a healthy heart. The nutrient-rich foods you eat on a whole-foods plant-based diet will also help reduce inflammation which has been shown to be an indicator for heart disease.

Prevent and Treat Type 2 Diabetes

Whole foods are naturally lower in sugar content. Even fruits that do contain sugar are packed with fiber and water so blood sugar levels don't spike. Studies have shown that switching to a diet that eliminates sugary foods and beverages will reduce the risk of type 2 diabetes. This diet also improves insulin resistance, a struggle for many who have diabetes.

Weight Loss

The whole-foods plant-based diet is filled with foods that are high in fiber, so you reduce the risk of overeating. You are also consuming more fresh fruits and vegetables that are lower in calories. When you are taking in fewer calories by eating plant-based foods, you will see weight loss occur.

Additionally, with a whole-foods plant-based diet you have complete control over what you consume. You do not need to worry about hidden carbs, sodium, fats, and sugars in the products you buy. Since there is an emphasis on creating all your own meals from scratch, from sauces to pasta, you know exactly what is going into everything you eat. When you have control over the ingredients, you know what is going in your food. There is less risk of unintentionally sabotaging your efforts for eating foods you think are better for you when they are not.

Feel More Energized

Those who stick with a whole-foods plant-based diet will feel less weighed down, bloated, and overstuffed after they eat. Eating more plant-based foods will allow you to eat until you are satiated. These foods are also easier to digest so less energy is being redirected to your digestive tract to process your foods. The energy that would typically go toward digestion can be dispersed to other systems and parts of the body. Since you will be providing the body with the nutrients it needs it will function better and you will feel more energized.

Cons

It takes more planning and preparation to stick with the whole-foods plant-based diet. Since you are cutting out time saver foods like prepackaged or pre-cooked foods you need to do the cooking yourself. You have to wash, cut, and cook all your vegetables and fruits which can be time-consuming. This extra time spent in the kitchen can be inconvenient to most, but when you plan for it you can save yourself time by preparing your food days in advance.

There is debate about whether a whole-foods plant-based diet can save you money with your grocery bills. Some people find they spend less because they stock up on whole beans and grains. Others find the prices of organic fruits and vegetables to be more than they can afford. If you factor in that you are saving money by cutting out more expensive items like red meats and poultry your grocery bill may be about the same. Learning how to grocery shop within a budget can be a challenge for many.

Getting Started

Remind yourself that it is ok to struggle on some days with your nutrition, especially at the beginning. A whole-foods plant-based diet is for the long-term. The more often you are able to get yourself back on track and make more nutritious choices the better you will feel.

Learn to cook in big batches. This allows you to get multiple meals out of what you are making without having to spend extra time in the kitchen. Your freezer will become your best friend on this diet. Make a second batch of any cooked meal you prepare and freeze it for weeks and sometimes months.

Don't let your fresh foods go to waste. If you have fruits and vegetables that are going to go bad before you have a chance to use them, freeze them. You can use fruits in smoothies and the vegetables can be used in a variety of ways.

You can even freeze cooked whole grains. When preparing meals you are serving with grains, make extra. You can portion the extra servings of grain out, store them in the freezer, and use them later. Extra grains can also be stored in the fridge and added to salads throughout the week.

Buying uncooked beans saves you money and they have a long shelf life. Uncooked beans do require extra prep time for soaking and cooking but you can use canned beans instead to save on time. Be sure to rinse and drain them thoroughly before heating them. You can also freeze leftover beans. Freezing extra cooked beans allows you to easily add the beans to many dishes like soups and stir fries.

Get creative and don't be afraid to try new things. On a whole-foods plant-based diet you want to add more flavors to your typical recipes. Try out new herbs and spices, and use food in a new way. Beans and cashews can be pureed to make into sauces. Your meals do not have to be bland and boring, but you do need to be open to try new flavors.

When possible, shop at your local farmers market. You will get better prices on your fresh fruits and vegetables and they are less likely to be sprayed with chemicals to preserve their freshness.

Find a milk alternative such as soy milk, almond milk, or oat milk. These items will provide you with the calcium you need and have the additional vitamin D necessary to absorb the calcium. This is true for zinc, iron, and B vitamins. Cutting back on animal products will decrease the amount of these minerals and vitamins. Incorporate plenty of beans, whole grains, and nutritional yeast into your meals as well.

7-Day Meal Plan

Monday

Breakfast: Steel-cut oats made with almond or soy milk topped with cinnamon, banana slices, and ground flax seed.

Snack: Apple slices and nut butter.

Lunch: Roasted beet salad with spinach and edamame.

Snack: Corn tortilla chips with fresh salsa or guacamole.

Dinner: Tofu stir-fry with brown rice (cook the brown rice in vegetable broth) served with snap peas, broccoli, spinach, and almond slices.

Tuesday

Breakfast: Tofu scramble with spinach, mushrooms, onion, and peppers wrapped in a whole-grain tortilla.

Snack: Fresh berries with coconut cream.

Lunch: Black bean burrito with mixed greens, tomatoes, onions, and peppers wrapped in a whole grain tortilla.

Snack: A handful of unsalted almonds.

Dinner: Chickpea curry served with a mixed green salad.

Wednesday

Breakfast: Quinoa breakfast bowl.

Snack: ¾ cup of edamame and an orange or clementine.

Lunch: Red lentil soup.

Snack: Avocado whole-grain toast.

Dinner: Apple pecan stuffed butternut squash and a side of mixed greens.

Thursday

Breakfast: Oats made with coconut milk, topped with fresh berries, shredded coconut, and walnuts.

Snack: An apple and half a cup of almonds.

Lunch: Black bean burger on a whole grain bun and baked sweet potato fries.

Snack: Celery sticks with nut butter.

Dinner: Vegan chili.

Friday

Breakfast: Breakfast Smoothie (blend together 1 cup of almond milk, 1 cup of kale, 1 cup of spinach, ½ cup of blueberries, 1 banana, 1 tablespoon of nut butter, and a drizzle of pure maple syrup).

Snack: Mixed fruit salad.

Lunch: Chopped vegetables (cabbage, celery, carrots, radish, broccoli, onions, and bell peppers) mixed with quinoa and drizzled with a turmeric dressing.

Snack: Black bean brownies.

Dinner: Chickpea or Black bean pasta with mushrooms and kale.

Saturday

Breakfast: Black bean burrito with avocado and tomatoes and a cup of fresh melon.

Snack: Tropical Smoothie (blend together a cup of almond milk, half a cup of pineapple, half a cup of strawberries, half a cup of mango, and half an avocado).

Lunch: Chipotle-lime cauliflower rice with black beans, mushrooms, and half an avocado (sliced).

Snack: Roasted red peppers and hummus on a slice of whole grain bread.

Dinner: Zucchini noodles with roasted brussel sprouts, mushrooms and spinach tossed in a cashew alfredo sauce.

Sunday

Breakfast: Breakfast Smoothie (blend together 1 cup of almond milk, ¼ cup of cashew butter, 1 banana, ½ cup of blueberries, ½ cup of kale, ½ cup of blackberries and a drizzle of pure maple syrup).

Snack: Fresh fruit and dairy-free yogurt.

Lunch: Stuffed sweet potato (stuff with kale, black beans, and sweet peppers) drizzled with a hummus dressing.

Snack: Roasted chickpeas.

Dinner: Grilled wild-caught salmon with cauliflower mash and roasted vegetables.

Chapter 20:

The Zone Diet

The zone diet does more than tell you what you should and should not eat, it provides you with a strategy to properly plan your meals. The diet is a steady approach to weight loss with most people losing about a pound a week. Those who may not have been successful with a restricted diet, calorie counting, or portion control may find the Zone diet to be a new and effective way to finally shed unwanted weight.

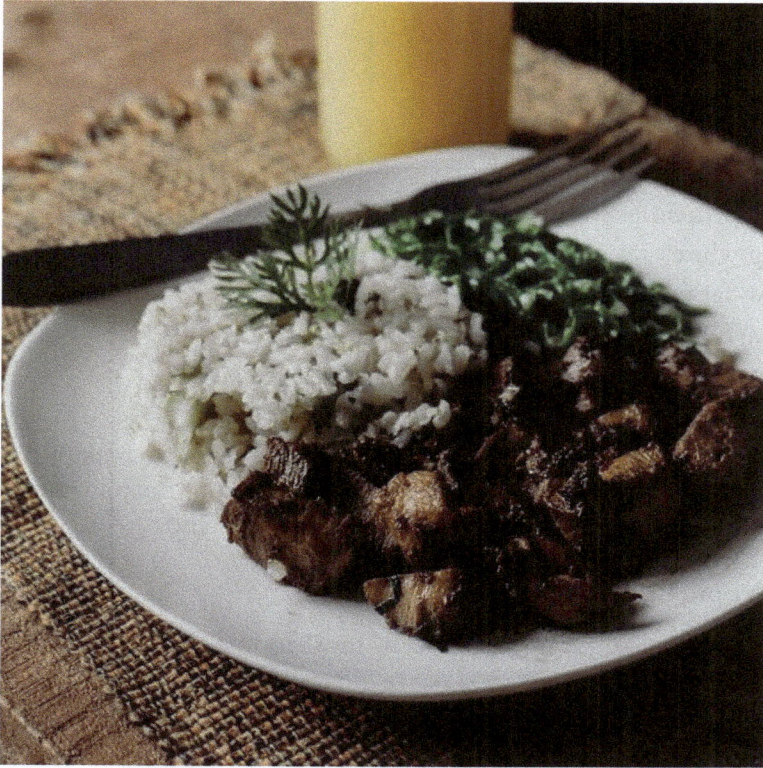

What Is the Zone Diet?

The Zone diet breaks meals down into three zones: low-fat protein, healthy fat, and carbs (non-starchy fruits and vegetables). The zones are further broken down into blocks which provide you with the suggested serving you should consume. Each day you should check off a certain number of blocks; women should consume 11 blocks a day and men should consume 14. The blocks are designed to ensure that each meal has a mix of the right macros. You won't be able to fill up on a large portion of carbs at lunch and then have a dinner that consists of a large portion of protein. This ensures you are eating a balanced diet throughout your day which provides your body with the right amount of energy to feel productive.

Protein block options include:

- lean beef or pork
- lamb, veal, or game
- fish and shellfish
- soy protein like tofu
- egg whites
- low-fat cheese
- low-fat milk
- low-fat yogurt

Each protein portion should equal around seven grams or make up a third of your plate. If you are eying this size, a portion of protein would be around the size and thickness of the palm of your hand.

Carb block options include:

- vegetables like peppers, spinach, mushrooms, cucumbers, and yellow squash
- chickpeas
- grains like oats and barley
- fruits like berries, oranges, plums, and berries

Each portion should average nine grams or make up two thirds of your plate. Try to choose carbs that are low on the glycemic index.

Fat blocks consist of:

- avocados
- nuts
- nut butter
- tahini
- oils like olive oil, sesame oil, and canola oil

Each portion should equal about one and a half grams. Monounsaturated fats should not be consumed.

Foods considered unfavorable on the Zone diet include:

- high-sugar fruits (dried fruits, mangoes, grapes, raisins, bananas)
- Starchy vegetables (corn, carrots, potatoes)
- refined and processed carbs (bread, pasta, white flour products)
- processed foods (muffins, breakfast cereals)
- foods with added sugar (cookies, cakes, candy)
- soft drinks

Unlike many of the other diets in this book, the Zone diet does incorporate calorie counting. Women should aim for about 1,200 calories a day while men aim for 1,500 calories. There are also more rules to follow, to the best of your ability. Some of these rules include:

- Eating within an hour of waking.
- Never go more than five hours without eating.
- Eat a snack before bedtime.
- Incorporate moderate and consistent exercise into your day.

These guidelines, along with the specific combination of protein, carbs, and fat, are designed to get you "in the zone." This diet takes into consideration three blood values; TG/HDL ratio, AA/EPA ratio, and HbA1c levels. When these levels are in a healthy range you are said to be "in the zone," meaning your body is using the foods you consume in an effective manner to function properly and provide you with consistent energy throughout the day. Let's go over these ratios in more detail.

TG/HDL represent the triglycerides (bad fat) to good cholesterol levels. When you have a low value your cholesterol is in good standing. The zone diet recommends a TG/HDL value of one as good. Anything high increases the risk of heart disease. Keep in mind that you cannot test your TG/HDL levels on your own. You need to go to a professional healthcare worker to get your cholesterol levels measured.

AA/EPA ratio looks at the levels of omega-6 fatty acids and omega-3 fatty acids in the body. If you have a low value your body contains more omega-3 fatty acids which helps reduce inflammation. The Zone diet encourages a level no higher than three. Higher AA/EPA levels have been linked to chronic disease, obesity, and depression. You can purchase a home kit to test your AA/EPA levels.

HbA1c represents the glycated hemoglobin in the body which shows your blood sugar levels. The Zone diet suggests you have a value of 5% or lower. Higher HbA1c levels puts you at greater risk for type two diabetes. Your HbA1c levels can only be checked by a health care professional and is typically checked regularly over a three month period to give the most accurate readings.

Even if you do not get these values tested you know you are in the zone when you feel an increase in energy and experience more mental focus throughout your day.

Benefits

The Zone diet ensures you are consuming the right balance of macros (protein, fat, and carbs), at each meal. While many other diets encourage a balance of these macros, most do not lay out an easy to follow plan to ensure that each meal has the right mix of these nutrients, For this reason, the Zone diet offers a range of benefits that may be similar but easier to achieve when compared to other diets.

Reduces Inflammation

Inflammation in the body increases when one consumes too much unhealthy fat and not enough or unbalanced macronutrients (fat, proteins, and carbohydrates). Individuals who eat a standard Western diet consume a high amount of unhealthy fats, processed carbs, and low-quality proteins. They also do not get the right balance of nutrients and consume far more omega-6 fatty acids over omega-3 fatty acids. Consuming more omega 6-fatty acids (found in vegetable oils) can increase blood pressure, put you at greater risk of blood clots, and cause you to retain excess water. High amounts of omega-6 fatty acids from eating fried foods and other meals cooked with processed vegetable oils also increase inflammation. A study published in the *Journal of the American College of Nutrition* indicates that the Zone diet can help reduce inflammation caused by nutrition. The study showed that a protein-rich, low-glycemic-index diet that also supplements omega-3 fatty acids reduces inflammation in individuals with type 2 diabetes (Stulnig, 2015). This study also showed that these individuals reduced their waistline and improved their glycemic levels.

Burns Fat for Weight Loss

You may not notice the scale move at first as your body burns up stored fat, but you will notice your clothes fit better and you may even need to go down a size or more. The diet is designed to burn fat even in the first weeks of being on it. Rapid weight loss on other diets typically reflects water weight or muscle mass loss; this weight usually is gained back quickly. The Zone diet on the other hand, provides essential nutrients the body needs while activating it to burn through the stored fat that can lead to poor health and obesity. The diet is also designed so that you lose weight at a steady pace, around one to two pounds a week. Though this may feel slow, this is a healthy and more effective way to lose unwanted pounds and keep the weight off.

Flexible

The diet is easy to adjust to your health goals. When trying to lose weight you craft your meals around-consuming fewer calories. Once you have reached your target weight you can increase your calorie intake to maintain your healthy weight. It is also easy to adjust your meal plans when or if you have an off day where you consume more calories than anticipated. There is no guilt or judgment around eating the foods you enjoy and the diet helps you learn to choose foods that are better for you more often.

The Zone diet can be beneficial to those who have tried and not had success with changing their diet in the past. It helps teach you a new way of eating. While there are many restrictions and guidelines to follow, each of these can help an individual recognize their body's hunger cues. When you are more in tune with your body you know how to better provide it with what it needs. Building a better relationship with food will naturally begin to feel better about what you eat, improve your health, and lose weight.

Cons

This diet has a lot more rules, can be overwhelming, and confusing. Meals need to follow many requirements. You need to eat from the appropriate blocks, track the times of your meals (including snacks), and count calories. This can be a lot to handle when you are trying to lose weight and get healthy. Those who have success on this type of diet need the clear cut rules; others will struggle with the limitation and directions to follow.

The Zone diet does not fall into a high-fat and protein diet as it keeps portions within the recommended range. Those with certain health conditions like kidney disease should consult a doctor before beginning the zone diet. Higher intake of fat and protein can also raise cholesterol levels which increases your chances of developing heart disease. It is important to monitor cholesterol levels especially if you are at higher risk for heart disease or already have high cholesterol.

The calorie restriction can cause you to feel hungry throughout the day. While your meals are balanced with filling foods, it is common for many to not feel full throughout the entire day. It takes time for your body to transition to the caloric intake and many people end up binging or overeating before giving their body the time to adapt. Remember, this is a long-term plan. If you have struggled with eating too much you can adjust the meal plan to include more of the low caloric, yet filling foods that will keep you on track.

Getting Started

Get a tracking system. Whether you use pen and paper, set up a note on your phone, or use a Zone Diet tracker, you want to have something in place to track your meals, calories, and times you eat. Once you have gotten used to the timing and portioning of your meals, you won't need to track as often. It can be incredibly useful to see what you eat and when to better plan your meals in the future when you begin this plan.

Plan your meals ahead of time. Planning out your meals will help you get used to the right portions and balance with each meal. You are less likely to get off track when you plan your meals and it simplifies the whole process.

Start your meals with low-fat protein, then move on to the rest of your plate. The protein will help you feel satiated sooner and the carbs will keep you feeling fuller for longer.

Plan your meals for every two and a half to four hours. Big meals should have about four hours in between them. If you are eating a snack, plan for another meal about two and half hours after your snack. Meals and snacks should not be skipped, even if you are not particularly hungry. Your day should consist of three meals and two snacks. Structure your meals so that 40% of your meal consists of healthy carbs, 30% consist of lean proteins, and 30% consist of healthy fats.

Always try to drink water with every meal. You should be aiming to drink eight eight-ounce glasses of water a day.

7-Day Meal Plan

Monday

Breakfast: Oatmeal with banana and cinnamon.

Snack: A hard-boiled egg and avocado slices on whole-wheat toast.

Lunch: Chicken and vegetable soup with a side of mixed greens.

Snack: Cottage cheese with fresh berries or peaches.

Dinner: Almond crusted chicken with roasted asparagus and steamed vegetables.

Tuesday

Breakfast: Spinach and mushroom omelet.

Snack: Smoothie (blend together a cup of almond milk, ½ cup of yogurt, a banana, ½ cup of spinach, a tablespoon flax seed, and half a cup of mixed berries).

Lunch: Brown rice bowl with black beans, salsa, and guacamole.

Snack: Carrots and bell pepper sticks with hummus.

Dinner: Lean steak and vegetable stir-fry.

Wednesday

Breakfast: Scrambled egg on whole-wheat toast with tomatoes, lettuce, and avocado.

Snack: Greek yogurt with walnuts and apple slices.

Lunch: Tuna salad (made with Greek yogurt) on whole-wheat toast and a side of mixed greens.

Snack: Poached pears.

Dinner: Turkey chili.

Thursday

Breakfast: Quinoa breakfast bowl with apples and cinnamon.

Snack: Cottage cheese and a cup of melon.

Lunch: Bone broth soup with a whole wheat roll and a side of mixed fruit.

Snack: Tuna salad and whole wheat crackers.

Dinner: Zucchini noodles with turkey meatballs.

Friday

Breakfast: Vegetable frittata and a side of sliced melon.

Snack: Oats and Berries Smoothie (blend together 1 ½ cups of almond milk, ¼ cup oats, ¼ cup greek yogurt, and 1 cup of mixed berries).

Lunch: Grilled chicken with lettuce, bell pepper, cucumber, and celery in a whole-wheat pita with a half cup of fresh strawberries.

Snack: Banana and apple slices with a tablespoon of almond butter on whole-wheat toast.

Dinner: Poached salmon with roasted cauliflower, asparagus, and sweet potato.

Saturday

Breakfast: Fruit, nuts, and yogurt parfait.

Snack: Tomato, cucumber, and mozzarella.

Lunch: Shrimp fried rice (with brown rice).

Snack: Nut butter, banana, and chia seed pudding.

Dinner: Grilled steak salad with a side of fresh cantaloupe.

Sunday

Breakfast: Breakfast burrito (eggs, black beans, and salad greens in a whole wheat tortilla) with a half cup of mixed fruit.

Snack: Smoothie (blend together a cup of almond milk, a cup of mixed berries, and a cup of spinach).

Lunch: Cabbage soup.

Snack: Hard boiled eggs and a piece of fruit.

Dinner: Chicken zucchini noodle pad thai.

Conclusion

Being stuck at a weight you are not comfortable or happy with does not have to be your permanent situation. Going from one disappointing fad diet to another is not the solution. You can choose a healthy diet that not only allows you to lose weight but can be adopted for life.

You now have 20 fantastic diets that will allow you to jumpstart your weight loss journey and set you on a path for a longer, healthier, and more energized life. Each of the diets mentioned in this book have its own unique approach to help you lose weight and keep it off. You just have to decide which approach best fits your lifestyle and will lead to the long-term results you desire.

One last thing I want to mention is the importance of exercise on your weight loss journey. As you have learned, not all the diets mentioned here require exercise, while others incorporate it into the plan. If you want to lose weight and keep it off, exercise is vital. However, incorporating exercise into your daily routine should be done in the same way you make changes to your diet. You do not need to start off exercising 30 minutes every day, especially if you do not exercise regularly already. Trying to go all in and commit to an exercise routine you know is going to be hard to maintain will only lead to skipping it or finding a way to avoid it all together. Exercise should be enjoyable and not a burden or tortuous activity you dread. You can find ways to incorporate a little more physical activity into your day or week by making small adjustments to things you already do.

The important thing is choosing an exercise routine you can manage for the long-term. It is better to start off with a short exercise routine that you know you can commit to than a routine you are going to be stressing over not having the time for. If you can only add in ten minutes of walking each day, then commit to that. Once you start feeling more fit and energized you can build on the routine you already created.

Remember, the key to lasting changes is consistency. Do not look at changing your eating habits and exercise routine as an all-or-nothing. make a few small changes you can commit to sticking with daily, then build from there. Even if you can only walk for five or ten minutes a day, as long as you stick with it every day you will feel better and see the weight come off and stay off. Create the habits for the healthy lifestyle you want to live and you will experience a lifetime of benefits.

Now you have a list of diets to help you lose weight and achieve optimal health. The only thing for you to do is get started. Choose the diet that is best for you, your goals, and your lifestyle. I wish you luck on your journey. I cannot wait for you to experience the slimmer, healthier, and more energized you!

References

Barnosky, A. R., Hoddy, K. K., Unterman, T. G., & Varady, K. A. (2014). Intermittent fasting vs daily calorie restriction for type 2 diabetes prevention: a review of human findings. *Translational Research, 164*(4), 302–311. https://doi.org/10.1016/j.trsl.2014.05.013

Bashinsky, R. (2020, March 4). *6 MIND Diet Recipes to Give Your Brain a Boost.* Health.com. https://www.health.com/food/mind-diet-recipes

Bellini, M., Tonarelli, S., Barracca, F., Morganti, R., Pancetti, A., Bertani, L., de Bortoli, N., Costa, F., Mosca, M., Marchi, S., & Rossi, A. (2020). A Low-FODMAP Diet for Irritable Bowel Syndrome: Some Answers to the Doubts from a Long-Term Follow-Up. *Nutrients, 12*(8). https://doi.org/10.3390/nu12082360

Bhandari, K. (2018, July 16). *Best detox drinks to lose weight fast, try green tea, mint, honey and more.* Hindustan Times. https://www.hindustantimes.com/fitness/best-detox-drinks-to-lose-weight-fast-try-green-tea-mint-honey-and-more/story-D8xtPwvjHOYQ7f7LCrM95M.html

Bjarmadottir, A. (2019, January 10). *Do detox diets and cleanses really work?* Healthline. https://www.healthline.com/nutrition/detox-diets-101#toxins

Brazier, Y. (2019, February 18). *What is the South Beach diet.* Medical News Today. https://www.medicalnewstoday.com/articles/7501#risks

Brazier, Y. (2020, April 27). *The raw food diet: Should I try it?* Medical News Today. https://www.medicalnewstoday.com/articles/7381

Buckingham, L. (2015, April 7). *How low-carb diets may be causing more kidney stones.* Daily Mail. https://www.dailymail.co.uk/health/article-3027906/How-low-carb-diets-causing-kidney-stones.html

Buckland, N. J., Camidge, D., Croden, F., Lavin, J. H., Stubbs, R. J., Hetherington, M. M., Blundell, J. E., & Finlayson, G. (2018). A Low Energy–Dense Diet in the Context of a Weight-Management Program Affects Appetite Control in Overweight and Obese Women. *The Journal of Nutrition, 148*(5), 798–806. https://doi.org/10.1093/jn/nxy041

Can eating a vegetarian diet really help you live longer? (n.d.). Sanitarium.com.au; Sanitarium Health & Wellbeing. https://www.sanitarium.com.au/health-nutrition/vegetarian-eating/eating-a-vegetarian-diet-can-help-you-live-longer#:~:text=A%20team%20of%20researchers%20at

Challa, H. J., Uppaluri, K. R., & Ameer, M. A. (2021, May 19). *DASH diet to stop hypertension.* Ncbi; StatPearls Publishing. https://www.ncbi.nlm.nih.gov/books/NBK482514/

Derbyshire, E. J. (2017). Flexitarian Diets and Health: A Review of the Evidence-Based Literature. *Frontiers in Nutrition, 3*, 55. https://doi.org/10.3389/fnut.2016.00055

Digestive Health Team. (2020, January 3). *Are You Planning a Cleanse or Detox? Read This First.* Health Essentials from Cleveland Clinic; Health Essentials from Cleveland Clinic. https://health.clevelandclinic.org/are-you-planning-a-cleanse-or-detox-read-this-first/

Dolson, L. (2020, February 18). *Everything to know about the three phases of the South Beach Diet.* Verywell Fit. https://www.verywellfit.com/what-to-expect-south-beach-diet-2242435

Editor. (2019, January 15). *Glycemic index (GI) and diabetes.* Diabetes.co.uk. https://www.diabetes.co.uk/diet/glycaemic-index-diet-and-diabetes.html

Fletcher, J. (2019, April 4). *Intermittent fasting for weight loss: 5 tips to start.* Medical News Today. https://www.medicalnewstoday.com/articles/324882#effects-on-exercise

Frey, M. (2020, January 17). *Pros and cons of the DASH diet.* Verywell Fit. https://www.verywellfit.com/dash-diet-pros-and-cons-3973825#toc-cons

Frey, M. (2021, January 28). *Getting started with a vegan diet.* Verywell Fit. https://www.verywellfit.com/vegan-diet-grocery-lists-and-more-4766952

Ghannoum, M., & Lansman, A. (n.d.). *How Does the Paleo Diet Affect Your Gut Microbiome?* BIOHM Health. https://www.biohmhealth.com/blogs/health/how-does-the-paleo-diet-effect-your-gut-microbiome

Groves, M. (2019, February 12). *The Mayo Clinic Diet Review: Does It Work for Weight Loss?* Healthline. https://www.healthline.com/nutrition/mayo-clinic-diet

Gunnars, K. (2018, August 2). *The Atkins diet: Everything you need to know.* Healthline. https://www.healthline.com/nutrition/atkins-diet-101#_noHeaderPrefixedContent

Gunnars, K. (2020, March 16). *5 Studies on the Mediterranean Diet — Does It Really Work?* Healthline. https://www.healthline.com/nutrition/5-studies-on-the-mediterranean-diet#TOC_TITLE_HDR_2

Gunnars, K. (2021, March 25). *6 Popular ways to do intermittent fasting.* Healthline. https://www.healthline.com/nutrition/6-ways-to-do-intermittent-fasting#TOC_TITLE_HDR_8

Gunnars, K., & Link, R. (2021, October 25). *Mediterranean Diet 101: Meal Plan, Foods List, and Tips.* Healthline. https://www.healthline.com/nutrition/mediterranean-diet-meal-plan#what-is-it

Halas-Liang, M. (2016, April 27). *Crohn's and the FODMAP elimination diet*. Inflammatory Bowel Disease. https://inflammatoryboweldisease.net/nutrition/crohns-and-the-fodmap-elimination-diet

Harvard Health Publishing. (2020, August 31). *Should you try the keto diet?* Harvard Health; Harvard Health. https://www.health.harvard.edu/staying-healthy/should-you-try-the-keto-diet

Jess. (n.d.). *114 little paleo diet tips that make a huge difference*. Paleo Grubs. https://paleogrubs.com/paleo-diet-guide/tips

Jönsson, T., Granfeldt, Y., Ahrén, B., Branell, U.-C., Pålsson, G., Hansson, A., Söderström, M., & Lindeberg, S. (2009). Beneficial effects of a Paleolithic diet on cardiovascular risk factors in type 2 diabetes: a randomized cross-over pilot study. *Cardiovascular Diabetology*, *8*(1), 35. https://doi.org/10.1186/1475-2840-8-35

Juraschek, S. P., Miller, E. R., Chang, A. R., Anderson, C. A. M., Hall, J. E., & Appel, L. J. (2020). Effects of Sodium Reduction on Energy, Metabolism, Weight, Thirst, and Urine Volume. *Hypertension*, *75*(3), 723–729. https://doi.org/10.1161/hypertensionaha.119.13932

Kim, M.-H., & Bae, Y.-J. (2015). Comparative Study of Serum Leptin and Insulin Resistance Levels Between Korean Postmenopausal Vegetarian and Non-vegetarian Women. *Clinical Nutrition Research*, *4*(3), 175–181. https://doi.org/10.7762/cnr.2015.4.3.175

Kohanmoo, A., Faghih, S., & Akhlaghi, M. (2020). Effect of short- and long-term protein consumption on appetite and appetite-regulating gastrointestinal hormones, a systematic review and meta-analysis of randomized controlled trials. *Physiology & Behavior*, *226*, 113123. https://doi.org/10.1016/j.physbeh.2020.113123

Kris, G. (2020, March 13). *5 Studies on the Paleo Diet — Does It Work?* Healthline. https://www.healthline.com/nutrition/5-studies-on-the-paleo-diet#limitations

Kubala, J. (2018, June 12). *21 Reasons to Eat Real Food.* Healthline. https://www.healthline.com/nutrition/21-reasons-to-eat-real-food#TOC_TITLE_HDR_23

Lee, W. (2021, February 16). *The South Beach Diet.* WebMD; WebMD. https://www.webmd.com/diet/a-z/south-beach-diet-what-it-is

Levitt, S., & Zelman, K. M. (2020, August 28). *The Zone diet.* WebMD. https://www.webmd.com/diet/a-z/zone-what-it-is

Levy, J. (2020, January 21). *The 4 steps of the volumetrics diet.* Dr. Axe. https://draxe.com/nutrition/volumetrics-diet/

Link, R. (2020, August 11). *Volumetrics Diet Review: Does It Work for Weight Loss?* Healthline. https://www.healthline.com/nutrition/volumetrics-diet#weight-loss

Loughrey, D. G., Lavecchia, S., Brennan, S., Lawlor, B. A., & Kelly, M. E. (2017). The Impact of the Mediterranean Diet on the Cognitive Functioning of Healthy Older Adults: A Systematic Review and Meta-Analysis. *Advances in Nutrition, 8*(4), 571–586. https://doi.org/10.3945/an.117.015495

Low FODMAP diet. (n.d.). Gastroenterology Consultants of San Antonio. https://www.gastroconsa.com/patient-education/irritable-bowel-syndrome/low-fodmap-diet/

Mayo Clinic Diet. (n.d.). US News. https://health.usnews.com/best-diet/mayo-clinic-diet

Mayo Clinic Staff. (2020a, May 6). *Atkins Diet: What's behind the claims?* Mayo Clinic. https://www.mayoclinic.org/healthy-lifestyle/weight-loss/in-depth/atkins-diet/art-20048485#:~:text=The%20Atkins%20Diet%20holds%20that

Mayo Clinic Staff. (2020b, November 18). *Can a low-carb diet help you lose weight?* Mayo Clinic. https://www.mayoclinic.org/healthy-lifestyle/weight-loss/in-depth/low-carb-diet/art-20045831

Mayo Clinic Staff. (2021, December 11). *Gluten-free diet.* Mayo Clinic. https://www.mayoclinic.org/healthy-lifestyle/nutrition-and-healthy-eating/in-depth/gluten-free-diet/art-20048530

Migala, J. (2021, October 25). *8 ways to follow the Mediterranean diet for better health.* Eating Well. https://www.eatingwell.com/article/16372/8-ways-to-follow-the-mediterranean-diet-for-better-health/

Morris, M. C., Tangney, C. C., Wang, Y., Sacks, F. M., Barnes, L. L., Bennett, D. A., & Aggarwal, N. T. (2015). MIND diet slows cognitive decline with aging. *Alzheimer's & Dementia, 11*(9), 1015–1022. https://doi.org/10.1016/j.jalz.2015.04.011

Morris, M. C., Tangney, C. C., Wang, Y., Sacks, F. M., Bennett, D. A., & Aggarwal, N. T. (2015). MIND diet associated with reduced incidence of Alzheimer's disease. *Alzheimer's & Dementia: The Journal of the Alzheimer's Association, 11*(9), 1007–1014. https://doi.org/10.1016/j.jalz.2014.11.009

Muinos, L. (2019, October 4). *Pros and cons of the Low-FODMAP diet.* Verywell Fit. https://www.verywellfit.com/low-fodmap-diet-pros-and-cons-4705955

Paddock, C. (2019, May 14). *DASH diet reduced heart failure risk "by almost half" in people under 75.* Medical News Today. https://www.medicalnewstoday.com/articles/325175

Paul. (n.d.). *Flexitarians.* Nutritionfacts.org. https://nutritionfacts.org/topics/flexitarians/#:~:text=Although%20flexitarians%20do%20live%20longer

Pearson, T. A., Mensah, G. A., Alexander, R. W., Anderson, J. L., Cannon, R. O., Criqui, M., Fadl, Y. Y., Fortmann, S. P., Hong, Y., Myers, G. L., Rifai, N., Smith, S. C., Taubert, K.,

Tracy, R. P., Vinicor, F., Centers for Disease Control and Prevention, & American Heart Association. (2003). Markers of inflammation and cardiovascular disease: application to clinical and public health practice: A statement for healthcare professionals from the Centers for Disease Control and Prevention and the American Heart Association. *Circulation*, *107*(3), 499–511. https://doi.org/10.1161/01.cir.0000052939.59093.45

Rajagopal, S. (n.d.). *Gluten-Free Diet: Is it right for me?* Johns Hopkins Medicine. https://www.hopkinsmedicine.org/health/conditions-and-diseases/celiac-disease/what-is-a-glutenfree-diet

Raman, R. (2017, April 4). *The Zone Diet: A complete overview.* Healthline. https://www.healthline.com/nutrition/zone-diet#TOC_TITLE_HDR_2

Roan, S. (2018, March 7). *DASH Diet Linked to a Lower Risk of Depression in Older Adults.* Everyday Health. https://www.everydayhealth.com/depression/dash-diet-linked-lower-risk-depression-older-adults/

Scott, J. R. (2021a, April 22). *What Is the Mayo Clinic Diet?* Verywell Fit. https://www.verywellfit.com/information-about-the-mayo-clinic-diet-review-3494734

Scott, J. R. (2021b, October 27). *What Is the volumetrics diet?* Verywell Fit. https://www.verywellfit.com/the-volumetrics-diet-what-you-need-to-know-3496210

Seaver, V. (2021, December 1). *30-Day low-carb meal plan: 1,200 Calories.* EatingWell. https://www.eatingwell.com/article/291554/30-day-low-carb-meal-plan-1200-calories/

Sleiman, D., Al-Badri, M. R., & Azar, S. T. (2015). Effect of Mediterranean Diet in Diabetes Control and Cardiovascular Risk Modification: A Systematic Review. *Frontiers in Public Health*, *3*, 69. https://doi.org/10.3389/fpubh.2015.00069

Sreenivas, S. (2021, September 27). *What to know about the MIND diet.* WebMD. https://www.webmd.com/alzheimers/what-to-know-about-mind-diet

Starting the low FODMAP diet. (n.d.). Monash University. https://www.monashfodmap.com/ibs-central/i-have-ibs/starting-the-low-fodmap-diet/

Stein, N. (2018, December 9). *Pros and cons of a vegetarian diet.* LIVESTRONG.COM. https://www.livestrong.com/article/196211-pros-cons-of-a-vegetarian-diet/

Stulnig, T. M. (2015). The ZONE Diet and Metabolic Control in Type 2 Diabetes. *Journal of the American College of Nutrition, 34*(sup1), 39–41. https://doi.org/10.1080/07315724.2015.1080110

Taub-Dix, B. (2019, January 3). *What is a flexitarian diet? What to eat and how to follow the plan.* Everyday Health. https://www.everydayhealth.com/diet-nutrition/diet/flexitarian-diet-health-benefits-food-list-sample-menu-more/

The T. Colin Campbell Center for Nutrition Studies. (2019, May 30). *Living a whole food, plant-based life.* Center for Nutrition Studies. https://nutritionstudies.org/whole-food-plant-based-diet-guide/

Torres, P. (2020, January 18). *Why low-carb diets aren't the answer.* The Healthy. https://www.thehealthy.com/weight-loss/why-low-carb-diets-arent-the-answer/

Tricò, D., Moriconi, D., Berta, R., Baldi, S., Quinones-Galvan, A., Guiducci, L., Taddei, S., Mari, A., & Nannipieri, M. (2021). Effects of Low-Carbohydrate versus Mediterranean Diets on Weight Loss, Glucose Metabolism, Insulin Kinetics and β-Cell Function in Morbidly Obese Individuals. *Nutrients, 13*(4), 1345. https://doi.org/10.3390/nu13041345

Turner-McGrievy, G. M., Davidson, C. R., Wingard, E. E., Wilcox, S., & Frongillo, E. A. (2015). Comparative effectiveness of plant-based diets for weight loss: A randomized controlled trial of five different diets. *Nutrition*, *31*(2), 350–358. https://doi.org/10.1016/j.nut.2014.09.002

U.S. Department of Health and Human Services. (2006). *Your Guide to lowering Your Blood Pressure With DASH*. https://www.nhlbi.nih.gov/files/docs/public/heart/new_dash.pdf

What is the Atkins diet, and is it healthy? (2021, January 5). Health Essentials from Cleveland Clinic. https://health.clevelandclinic.org/what-is-the-atkins-diet-and-is-it-healthy/

Winters, N. (2020, December 5). *11 significant health benefits of the ketogenic diet*. KETO-MOJO. https://keto-mojo.com/article/top-11-health-benefits-of-keto/#

Image References

Arledge, K. (2019, October 30). [Chicken and green beans] {digital image}. Retrieved from Unsplash. https://unsplash.com/photos/V7hibs9xhe4

Bluebird Provisions (2020, December 9). [Bone broth in white bowls on cutting board with vegetables] {digital image}. Retrieved from Unsplash. https://unsplash.com/photos/WPaUC6FrAZ0

Cocobols. (2020, September 23). [Coconut bowl full of fresh spring rolls] {digital image}. Retrieved from Unsplash. https://unsplash.com/photos/zW8wA4QwS2M

Dahl, A. (2016, October 14). [Steak salad] {digital image}. Retrieved from Pixabay https://pixabay.com/photos/steak-salad-sunt-1735136/

Daniels, K. (2019, June 6). [A platter of veggies, fruits, nuts, and seeds. Whole 30 approved] {digital image}. Retrieved from Unsplash. https://unsplash.com/photos/DdB-4uOJNVA

Golovac, A. (2018, August 15). [Green goddess pita] {digital image}. Retrieved from Unsplash. https://unsplash.com/photos/MAbhhj3QCXQ

Hansen, R. (2019, July 25). [Mixed fruits] {digital image}. Retrieved from Unsplash. https://unsplash.com/photos/_WpB9l8_Kn4

Kolodzoejczak, K. (2021, February 19). [Vegan dinner] {digital image}. Retrieved from Unspalsh. https://unsplash.com/photos/ue1WvpHlccI

Lee, C. (2016, June 27). [Meal with salmon and zucchini] {digital image}. Retrieved from Unsplash. https://unsplash.com/photos/awj7sRviVXo

Mory, A. (2018, September 21). [Grilled meat, rice, and greens] {digital image}. Retrieved from Unsplash. https://unsplash.com/photos/O4CVzHODjjM

Munsell, A. (2015, May 20). [Steak dinner] {digital image}. Retrieved from Unsplash. https://unsplash.com/photos/auIbTAcSH6E

Olsson, E. (2018, October 30). [Bread toasts with avocado, banana, tomato] {digital image}. Retrieved from Unsplash. https://unsplash.com/photos/2IxTgsgFi-s

Olsson, E. (2018, November 27). [Plant-based meal prep] {digital image}. Retrieved from Unsplash. https://unsplash.com/photos/lMcRyBx4G50

Pelzer, A. (2017, December 7) [Vegan salad bowl] {digital image}. Retrieved from Unsplash. https://unsplash.com/photos/IGfIGP5ONV0

Photo Mix-Company (2016, July 21). [Lime drink] {digital image} Retrieved from Pixabay. https://pixabay.com/photos/drink-glass-lime-mint-cold-fresh-1532300/

Primeau, N. (2018, October 24) [Veggie salad] {digital image}. Retrieved from Unsplash. https://unsplash.com/photos/-ftWfohtjNw

RitaE (2018, April 13) [Vegetable skewer] {digital image}. Retrieved from Pixabay. https://pixabay.com/photos/vegetable-skewer-paprika-tomato-3317060/

RitaE (2017, March 23). [Asparagus and steak] {digital image} Retrieved from Pixabay. https://pixabay.com/photos/asparagus-steak-veal-steak-veal-2169305/

RitaE (2016, April 5). [Asparagus, egg, and tomato] {digital image} Retrieved from Pixabay. https://pixabay.com/photos/meal-asparagus-dish-food-1307604/

Taylor, D. (2018, May 8). [Orange chicken, broccoli, and white rice] {digital image}. Retrieved from Unsplash. https://unsplash.com/photos/jFu2L04tMBc

www.ingramcontent.com/pod-product-compliance
Lightning Source LLC
Chambersburg PA
CBHW060037030426
42334CB00019B/2360